CHEMO THIS!

*Finding Your Balance & Creating
a Pathway Through Cancer*

*Wishing you good health
and good balance
in your life*

by

PATRICIA McBAIN-ROBERTS

P. McBain-Roberts

July 28, 2001.

Published by

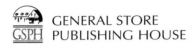 GENERAL STORE
GSPH PUBLISHING HOUSE

Box 28, 1694B Burnstown, Ontario, Canada K0J 1G0
Telephone (613) 432-7697 or 1-800-465-6072

ISBN 1-894263-37-5
Printed and bound in Canada

Design layout by Derek McEwen
Printing by Custom Printers of Renfrew Ltd.
Cover Artwork by Tim Yearington

General Store Publishing House
Burnstown, Ontario, Canada
©Copyright P. McBain-Roberts

Canadian Cataloguing in Publication Data

McBain-Roberts, P. (Patricia), 1951-
  Chemo this! : finding your balance and creating a pathway
through cancer

ISBN 1-894263-37-5

  1. McBain-Roberts, P. (Patricia), 1951-
  2. Breast-Cancer–Psychological aspects.
  3. Breast-Cancer–Patients–Ontario–Biography. I. Title.

RC280.B8M22 2001   362.1'9699449'0092   C2001-900025-1

This book is dedicated with love
to my mother
Onetta Mary Herbert Clark,
a breast cancer survivor
on her 80th birthday

Foreword

In *Chemo THIS!* Pat McBain-Roberts has well accomplished her goal of sharing her personal experience with breast cancer and giving us a valuable road map to help others who have to make this difficult journey. Her insights and advice are practical, highly applicable and from the heart.

The chapter written by her spouse, Bruce, is most relevant to family and friends wanting to be of support, but will also help others with cancer gain some insight into how much their illness affects everyone, particularly those close to them.

Pat writes with humour, a very necessary tool in the armamentarium of the battle with cancer. Though everyone's journey and experiences are unique, we can all find help along the path from those who have gone before, left footprints and cleared away some of the impediments. Pat's book gives us all such a guide. Everyone from cancer victims to caregivers, family and friends will find wisdom in these pages.

For me personally it was illuminating to see how the medical system is perceived, its limitations, its pitfalls and how each individual along the way can make a difference (for better or for worse). Thanks, Pat, for using your unfortunate experience as an opportunity for learning, personal growth and sharing so as to ease the way for those who follow.

Dr. Margaret Paul
General Surgeon

Table of Contents

Acknowledgements

Writing a book is like weaving a colourful tapestry. Here and there are people who bring precious threads of silver and gold to contribute to the process making the tapestry that much more exquisite. There are many people to thank for my safe journey and you will read about them in this book. There are a few who have contributed to the actual literary outcome and I want to say a special "thank you" for their involvement.

I wish to acknowledge the artful work of my editor, Jane Karchmar. It is Jane who initially recognized this book as a worthy project and it is Jane who has dotted the i's and crossed the t's and helped me to stick with the details long after I thought I was finished. Thank you for your partnership and your professional polish.

Lynn Johnston has provided her special cartoon from *For Better or For Worse*—a gift that will add to the smiles in this story. Her personal phone call to my home, her interest in supporting survivors of breast cancer, and the surprise offer to contribute her work are very much appreciated.

And to my astute and literate dear friend, Lynda Smith, thank you for the chatty Saturday afternoon lunches and the avid reviews of my early drafts. Lynda sharpened her pencil, asked me questions, made suggestions and nudged me forward.

I wish to thank Dr. Margaret Paul for taking the time from her demanding schedule to read my manuscript. Her confidence in this work and her straightforward feedback mean a great deal to me. Dr. Paul's trust that this story will make an important contribution to the medical community and the travelers who make this journey is the best reward of all.

Introduction

"Chemo This!" What an irreverent title for such a serious and life changing experience! My encounter with cancer has been an incredible journey of discovery that leaves me humbled and wiser. It has touched the lives of everyone in my family. And, at times, it has taken us to the darkest side of fear and anxiety.

My husband had been encouraging me to write this book since the beginning of this whole experience. One Sunday morning I said, "Well, if I *did* write a book, what should we call it?" I said "we" because we are partners in all things. He contemplated that notion for a few minutes over his coffee. Then he looked at me with a slight grin and quietly said with his customary dry humour, "How about '**Chemo THIS!**'"

That shot a laser beam right through my funny bone. We both laughed until I thought we would cry. "Oh no," I said, once I recovered my senses. I was horrified! "We couldn't do that, it's far too irreverent." But for the rest of the day, I broke into a fit of giggles every time it crossed my mind. Two weeks later, I was still chuckling. I decided, what the heck: I have cancer and it's my book. One thing I've noticed is that cancer has altered my view of what is significant in life. If my book's title made me smile, why would I hesitate? If we can't have some humour in this world, where would we all be?

The title stems from a species of "black humour" that often develops through such an experience. Cancer patients and those close to them inevitably begin to laugh with each other about the most serious and depressing aspects of their journey. It helps to alleviate the tension and builds a bond between compadres and soulmates.

At the time of this writing, the latest statistic is that one in eight Canadian women and one in nine American women will be diagnosed with breast cancer over their lifetime. That's staggering—a bloody epidemic by any stretch of the imagination! When I think of the lives that will be touched along with the cancer patients—the husbands, the sons, the daughters, the mothers and fathers, the coworkers and friends—I see an exponential impact and the need to help people get from one side of this to the other. I want to stretch out my hand and take these people from the fear of the unknown to a better understanding of what could transpire along the way. But all that being said, each person's journey will be unique and each individual will have to become the architect of his or her own pathway.

This book is not an attempt to provide medical facts as the main menu. Nor is it intended to be a book of "woe is me." It describes the discoveries I have made on my journey. It provides some very useful resources and insights that I have uncovered after an exhaustive flurry of research and a personal internal struggle to find some answers. My discoveries helped me to build my own pathway through cancer. I found a better balance between my professional and personal life. And I found something else along the way, something very special that I had never realized I was looking for. But I can't give away too many secrets just yet.

I recommend that you take advantage of the planning tool at the back of this book to capture your own ideas, as you find the keys that were helpful to me. My discoveries are woven throughout this story. But that's not all. There will be many of your own revelations.

Many people have written about the experience of having breast cancer. My greatest wish in writing this book is to share my own experience in the hope that some of my insights will help those who will walk this road in the days ahead. I don't know what my own future is to be. I do know that, regardless of the outcome, it has become even more important to me to leave a mark in the world that will help others. I have been to many places through this journey, all within an entirely different solar system of my mind. I have learned things that must be shared. To paraphrase Dr.

Bernie Siegel (1992), in *Meditations for Overcoming Life's Stresses and Strains:*

> *"You have a mountain to climb. Along the way there will be resources to help you. Feel free to use them. And when you get to the top, take the time to leave a note for those who will follow you . . ."*

Patricia McBain-Roberts

Chapter 1

The Cliff's Edge

I was oblivious to the Christmas season unfolding around me. The last time I had taken any notice of the outside world was when the slate gray of November had freeze-dried the countryside, leaving it dark and naked—in limbo. Our once lush forest had been turned to black stands of frozen sticks. It would be some time before winter's beauty would descend with a velvety layer of pristine snow. It was enough to make you want to curl up in a ball and pull the flannelette sheets up over your head.

Cancer was not on my agenda. It wasn't on my primary agenda, my secondary agenda or even my rainy day agenda. I was busy. I didn't have time for it and that was that. I have always been the "master of my own destiny." That clearly qualified me to be in full control of my own agenda planning.

The lump was only about the size of a tiny pearl. I could feel it as I ran the soap over my breast one morning in the shower. I ran my fingers back over it again. I must be imagining things. No one ever told me that a lump would feel like this, and I hadn't asked. A lump should feel more like a big grape, shouldn't it? The very word "lump" sounds large to me. I dismissed it. I had a lot to do that day in my role as a consultant. There were places to go, people to see and conference calls to make. My mind went to the activities of the upcoming day and swept me away. I loved my work. It was fascinating and I was totally consumed by it.

The next time I took a shower, I checked back into the "pearl site." It was gone. Thank goodness for that! I worry too much. Had I truly felt it or had it just been my imagination? I settled for imagination

1

and decided I wouldn't think about it anymore, because after all, cancer was *not* on my agenda. I made a point not to check my breast again for some time. That was quite a scare. I didn't want to get an upset like that again.

Eight years before, I had been sent for the first mammogram of my life. I was only forty years old, but the history of breast cancer in my family prompted the suggestion from my doctor. I complied with this as a routine checkup, just as I always had with my annual pap test. These things don't ruffle me. I have no interest in being sick and, therefore, I don't get sick. However, for some reason I feel the need to be a good patient and to comply with my doctor's requests. My mother taught me early in life to be very respectful of the medical profession. It's gently but deeply ingrained.

I have always been a healthy person, but I'm the only one in my family who can make that claim. At a very early age I adopted the role of "the healthy one" who would go on to have a normal life. My father was a fine but troubled soul who died of colon cancer at age seventy-three. I loved him dearly. My brother and sister, both older than I, were severely developmentally handicapped. My mother had delicate health much of her life, complicated by the sadness of family sickness and then her own breast cancer at age sixty. And then there was me—the healthy one, the self-appointed normal one—the lucky one.

That first mammogram didn't turn out to be routine. The radiologist found an abnormality that he thought should be checked further. We were sent off to a hospital in a much larger centre south of us, a four-hour journey from our hometown. My husband Bruce, my best friend, took me there and I was glad he was with me. We were moderately worried.

A biopsy was done and the verdict indicated the abnormality was benign. Good news. My mother's breast cancer had surfaced ten years before, along with the need for a radical mastectomy. I knew that a lot of female relatives on both the maternal and paternal sides of my family had also had breast cancer. Genetics, you know. Not a good prognosis for me. But genetics didn't mean a lot to me, because after all I was a solidly healthy specimen. I couldn't have told you exactly which relatives had experienced breast cancer, because I didn't listen all that closely to conversations about sickness.

So there it was: BENIGN, and proof once again that sickness did not have to be on my agenda. My breast was black and blue for a few days around the incision site. I slept for forty-eight hours and was back at work in three days. The world continued on. It was a relatively minor interruption in our lives.

Three weeks later, I had a call from the surgeon who had done the biopsy. It seemed that further study of the tissue now indicated that the cells were pre-cancerous. What a curious word, "pre-cancerous." What was that supposed to mean? "In essence," the doctor explained, "the surgeon removed cells that *might* one day have become cancerous." So it was all very good news. At least I thought it might be. I told Bruce. He was confused as well.

It wasn't until about a year later, when I asked my family doctor to complete some life insurance papers for me, that I discovered he had that word "cancer" on my history. The insurance rates tripled! I was very annoyed. I did NOT have cancer! I went to see him, and he informed me that yes indeed I had had cancer. I told my husband, who responded predictably, " But I thought the cells were *pre*-cancerous." My sentiments exactly! We puzzled over it and worried about it. But the cells had been removed and the problem was resolved. No follow-up treatment had been recommended, except to return to the centre for a yearly mammogram and checkup with the specialist.

My family doctor suggested one day that, given my family history, I should consider having my breasts removed. I was appalled and indignant. I quickly retorted, "A bus could run me over someday, too; that doesn't mean I should consider having my head removed, just in case." He looked wounded. So much for my mother's lessons in medical etiquette! I was angry about that suggestion for a long, long time and dismissed my doctor as being "overly zealous." Sheeeeeeesh!

Eight years went by. I had my mammogram faithfully every year. After about six years, it became a begrudging exercise. I began to think that if nothing had happened by now, it probably wouldn't. I was becoming more and more convinced that it must have been an overly cautious measure, and the worry slipped away. Or perhaps it was decidedly cancelled out.

This year, my annual appointment for a mammogram was scheduled for November 30, with a local doctor this time, at my request. I was tired of having to travel so far away to the specialist on a wild goose chase every year. The local doctor recommended by my family doctor was a surgeon. I was suspicious about that, not having forgotten his earlier recommendation, but I went along with it. I showed up promptly on time for the appointment. The doctor had been called out unexpectedly to surgery. I was miffed, but suppressed my reaction. I was a very busy person and this appointment had caused me to leave an important management meeting that I had wanted to attend. The doctor's assistant was very apologetic. She looked as if she was going to cry when her eyes glanced at the stack of patient files that would now have to be rebooked into an already impossible schedule. It seemed like a regular occurrence. I left without rebooking. Health care in our part of the world was in a disastrous state. Our doctors were severely overworked and the patients just kept lining up. I tried to be understanding.

By Christmas, the lump was back. It was in the same spot where I had originally discovered it. It was bigger this time. I said nothing to anyone. The lump continued to be there in the same spot every day. I was worried. Maybe I had cancer after all. I called to rebook my appointment for a checkup and mammogram with the recommended surgeon. The soonest I could get in was February, so that would have to do.

One night I dreamed that I was climbing up a very steep rock cliff. It was the middle of the night, rain was pouring down, and thunder and lightning were crashing all around me. The ocean waves were smashing against the cliff wall below. There was a damp cold that went right through to my bones. I was climbing on a narrow, winding pathway, trying with all my strength to get to the top of the cliff. When I finally reached the top, I found a massive white building that looked from the outside to be some sort of scientific observatory, with a very large dome open to the sky. I entered the building. They were expecting me. There was a group of scientists, working quietly and purposefully to prepare for my visit. No one looked up or spoke to me. The next thing I knew, I was lying naked on a table. The table began to move into an upright position and I was being immersed in a transparent tank of blue water. My whole body was to be covered in water. I understood that I would be there for some time. It did not frighten me. I was not concerned about breathing, but I was awake and aware of the entire procedure. I was cognizant of the fact that I had cancer, and that the scientists would have to conduct this complex procedure. When I awoke in the morning, I dismissed the dream as a mere unconscious symbol of my fears.

As the weeks passed, I became overwhelmed with what having cancer would mean to me, to my wonderful family and to my work that I loved so much. I had been working as a self-employed freelance consultant. I had independently arranged a good drug and hospital plan when I left an eleven-year tenure with the government, but no disability insurance. Why would I need to spend money for disability insurance when I was the master of my own destiny and could control my own health, as any omnipotent sort of being would do?

So here we were. Bruce, my spouse of only ten years was retired and on a well-deserved pension after thirty-two years of service with his employer. I had twin teenage boys preparing for university within the year. A number of years as a sole support parent had precluded a good financial plan for university fees for my two sons. And then there was a healthy mortgage payment each month and no disability insurance to cover my wages if I had to go into hospital. So, omnipotent one, what now?

I had no answers. My thoughts were like a dark, silent vacuum.

I had mastered a lot of difficult challenges in my life. Three radical career changes, the ending of two marriages that were never meant to be, and the death of my daughter, Robin, in her eighteenth year. Recreating my life from scratch through each of these transitions had not been easy. It wasn't something I talked about. I knew that each challenge had been an impossible mountain that I had managed to pull myself up and over, one small step at a time. Slipping into the cavern of no recovery had been a very real threat on more than one occasion. But I made it each time, and possibly that is where I became so firmly convinced that I could create any destiny for myself if I wanted badly enough to do it.

I became quite withdrawn in the month of January. My conversation was minimal. It wasn't unusual behaviour for me, at least not at home. I was often preoccupied with my work. My family had become quite accustomed to talking to me and realizing that I was answering them, but not really there. I was on automatic pilot. No one noticed and I was able to cover up my secret. I couldn't tell anyone because I just didn't know what the solution was. I had always been so good at helping other people to solve their problems. Until now, I had managed to resolve the difficult challenges that emerged in my own life. But this time was different. I had nothing to offer in the way of a remedy. The longer I could keep my secret, the less time my family would need to worry. Moments of conversations with my family seemed to slip into slow motion, like a "pause" on a video, captured in my memory in case there would not be many more. A smile, or an expression on the face of a loved one became precious treasures.

I went to sleep at night thinking about my sons and Bruce and even the dog being turned out of their own home. I was destitute. No matter how much I tried, I couldn't think of a resolution.

Slowly, it became evident to me that the only way out of this mess was to die. I would say nothing to anyone and I would die of breast cancer. Well, I suppose everyone has to die of something someday; I just hadn't ever considered that it would be so soon—my agenda, you know. At least I had life insurance and mortgage insurance. That would solve everything.

Did I want to die? Most assuredly not. I had everything in the world to live for. Bruce was the dearest partner any woman could ever want. I was thirty-six years old and had kissed a few toads before I found him. I had two beautiful, healthy twin boys just beginning their life's adventure. As fraternal twins, they had been a fascinating study in distinct but very special opposites. One wanted to become a computer engineer and was likely CEO material, while the other enthusiastically aspired to be ordained in the priesthood, or perhaps trained in social work. I wondered enviously what it would be like to watch all that play out for my boys. I finally had a modest but lovely home that I felt very comfortable in. And I had a fascinating job that I had wanted to do all my life. Even our dog, Woody, was a perfect, lovable creature that no one would deliberately say goodbye to.

My mother would be shattered—she had already had so much sadness. My brother might suffer a broken heart—he adored me. My stepdaughter had just encountered her first experience with death—her grandfather. It was devastating to her and I didn't want to add to her distress. My sister, who had been institutionalized all her life and didn't know me, or anyone else for that matter, would be the only soul not to feel the impact of my death.

But dying was my only solution. This challenge was not within my ability to control. I was defeated, powerless and bound to silence. In the past, I had always talked every trouble over with my spouse. He was my deep kindred spirit. He never failed to have a peaceful and helpful impact on me when life became impossible. He would say to me quietly, "This too shall pass." But not this time. There were no words of wisdom, no warm hugs that could make this go away. And I didn't want to burden him with the sadness that I was feeling. My love for him, on every dimension, was as deep as it could possibly be.

The lump was still there when January became February. Because a Calgary conference date conflicted with my doctor's appointment, I rescheduled my doctor to March 1st. I sensed that I was walking toward the edge of a very steep cliff and that the fall, when it happened, would be excruciating. I wasn't in a hurry to get to this unique spot in my life; I knew what my choices were.

Time at the Calgary conference was very troubling. There was an overwhelming amount of work to be thought out and implemented for the international firm I worked with. They were in the middle of one of the country's largest business mergers and I was to be an important stabilizing influence in my local area. A lot of people would be counting on me to help them through a terrifying time in their lives. Many employees with life-long careers in this company were to be moved into early retirement. People felt they were being pushed aside through restructuring like obsolete machinery. It was a difficult time for them.

The responsibility of the entire world seemed to be on my shoulders. And I was dying.

But one very positive thing happened on that trip. Our team of freelance consultants was given a verbal job offer to become core employees, rather than temporary contractors. That was something we had all been very interested in. But it quickly became another burden in my mind. Would they want me if they knew I had cancer? Was I to lose this wonderful job opportunity now, because of this deviation in my agenda? I cried myself to sleep a lot when I was at that conference. I was so very tired, probably dangling by a very thin thread of burnout and so many problems to think about for myself and the people that I loved and cared about. What a fine mess I was in this time!

Chapter 2

So What Does The Dog Have To Do With This?

It wasn't long before our dog, Woody, was onto my secret. His ninety pounds of black angora-like fur would lie on the floor across the room from me, studying every move I made, listening to every word I was thinking. Silent Sam, I liked to call him. I had always had a special focused attention from him in the mornings, when I was getting ready to face the day. But that was the only time. He would lie on the floor by my side and watch as I curled and brushed my hair, applied my mascara and lipstick. There was something about the rhythmic motions I was going through that made him feel peaceful. He knew the exact signals when the process was to conclude. Then he would rise to his feet in anticipation, prance around joyously, ready to usher me downstairs to join Bruce for his morning outing in the car.

From the time we had adopted him as a pup, Woody had always had a special attachment to my spouse, who had a gentle way with animals and people. Woody's attention was usually focused on his master, although he had enough affection to share with the rest of us. But there was a special bond between Woody and Bruce, who seemed to have a magical gift; the "dog whisperer," I called him. Woody was a wonderful addition to our family.

Woody had the ability to enchant anyone. He loved to put his head out the window when we were out for a drive, sniffing the air and letting his ears fly with wild abandon. Grownups who were looking far too serious as they stood on the street would grin involuntarily as we drove by. Little children would point and shout "woof, woof!" to see if they could get him to respond. Sometimes grown-up fellas in their trucks would do the same. I found this particularly comical. Our dog seemed to bring out the kid in everyone.

When we would go for an evening walk with Woody, it was rare to come home without at least one person having stopped to ask us delightedly, "What kind of dog is HE? Is he just a puppy?" And we would respond for the millionth time, "He is six years old but has a perpetual puppy face and he is a cross between a Newfoundland and a Flat Coat Retriever." And we would walk on, knowing that Woody had touched yet another life, if only for a brief moment.

One evening during my troubled, lonely period, Woody came over to me and put his sleek black face in my lap, rolled his eyes slowly upward and looked directly and deeply into my eyes. He'd been studying me again. It was a very understanding, sympathetic look. He was telling me that he knew my secret—he had read my thoughts. From that point onward, he began to sleep by my side of the bed. During the day, he frequently came to my side, but not for the usual tactile attention that he craved. He was running his own diagnostics, checking me over, telling me that everything was going to be all right. I sometimes wondered to myself if it was possible for animals to carry a human spirit inside them. Once in a while I would fleetingly think that my daughter's spirit might be within him. There was just an uncanny sense of his being incredibly wise and knowing, beyond any living creature's capacity.

I don't know how Woody knew that I was in trouble. I just know that he did and I doubted it not for a minute. He was a truly special and comforting friend.

About four days prior to my medical appointment with the recommended surgeon, I spontaneously made an appointment with my family doctor to show him the lump. I don't know what prompted me to do that, except to say that it was a turning point. My thinking had taken on a new dimension. Solutions were trying desperately to take shape. They weren't very good solutions, but somewhere a speck-of-a-seed-of-hope was forming.

I had some money set aside in mutual funds for my retirement. I hadn't considered this option before, because that money had always been firmly untouchable in my planning, that agenda of mine again. But now things were different. There was a more immediate need. It

didn't seem feasible that I could just stay quiet about my cancer and
rot away like some old ship. It occurred to me that there would have
to be a dying period—I couldn't just neatly shut off the switch and not
be any trouble to anyone. It was beginning to dawn on me that
perhaps if I tried, I might not die at all. I didn't want to go. Not yet.

If I were to tap into my mutual funds, at least that would keep
things glued together for my family. Perhaps we wouldn't have to lose
our home. Perhaps that first year of tuition could be paid for the first
departing son and his life planning toward university would not have to
be destroyed. I could think about plans for the second departing son
when I was well again. Thank goodness they were graduating a year
apart.

It was time to confide in my husband. I couldn't keep this from
him any longer. "I have a lump in my breast," I announced one
evening. He was quiet. I asked him to feel it, thinking that I needed to
prove it as medical fact. He knew that I sometimes worried over
needless things. Maybe he would think this was the case this time, as
well. He was a much calmer person than I. I could see the concern on
his face when he felt the lump, which now seemed to have grown to
the size of a large Italian olive. I reassured him that I was going to the
doctor the next day, and Bruce said he would take me to the
appointment. I was glad of that.

My family doctor readied himself for the routine breast exam.
He looked concerned when I told him of the lump. "Is it the same
breast where you had the biopsy eight years ago?" he asked quickly.
His fingers moved carefully in circular motions across every inch of
my breast. When he touched the lump in the outside quadrant of my
breast, he pulled back quickly from me. "Well, that's very OBVIOUS
and very HARD," he stated. He looked at me sharply and said no
more. I was filled with guilt. I told him that I had just found it two
weeks before. His silence indicated that he knew different. I felt
ashamed for having made that statement.

"I want to send a letter with you to the surgeon," he said. I
agreed to pick it up the next day. It was sealed. I held it up to the light
of the window but managed only to confirm the confidentiality of the
envelope that enclosed these writings about me. It probably is a letter
to tell her how much in denial I have been about my potential for

breast cancer, I grumbled inwardly. Denial. Yes, I had been in denial, I thought. How odd! I understand completely what denial is; I have read extensively about it. I have even taught the staff that I work with about denial. And yet here I was—the Number One Denial Offender. My doctor must have been very frustrated. All his concern and warnings had gone unheeded. I hadn't looked after myself as religiously as I should have and I knew it. I had a sedentary lifestyle, I wasn't as careful about my diet as I had been after the first scare. I was working myself to death, night and day and ready to drop from exhaustion. Well, four days to go and I would be on my surgeon's doorstep.

She read the letter from my family doctor. I watched her very closely to see if she would recognize me as the "denial offender." No luck—she had a poker face. She conducted her exam and then asked me to get dressed. When she returned, she began to draw a picture of a breast, indicating the ducts and nipple, and methodically explained the seriousness of my situation. She was very businesslike but not judgmental. It was such a relief to me, not to be judged. It was a bad sign, she said, that the lump was in the same breast that had caused concern eight years ago. It was also a bad sign that breast cancer was so prevalent in my family history. The lump was very hard, and her educated guess was that there was a 99% chance that it was cancerous. I knew from the look on her face and the words she was using, that she had it precisely. Her quiet, thoughtful approach spelled absolute competence. I had no question about this. She recommended surgery as soon as possible and offered three options:

- A biopsy with a week to wait to see if anything further was required;
- A lumpectomy and possibly chemotherapy or radiation, depending on the results;
- A mastectomy, to have my complete breast removed, with follow-up of chemo and/or radiation.

In a matter of thirty seconds, I agreed to sign a form that would allow a mastectomy, if she felt it the best option, once into the lump site. After three months of indecision, I knew that I couldn't fool around anymore. I am by nature a very decisive person. My nature was coming back to me with all this straight talk. But she encouraged me to take the form home, think it over and discuss it with my husband.

I went out to the car and told my kindred spirit the full story. I could tell by the look on his face that he knew we were in for a bad time. He needed time to reflect on all this before I would know his thoughts. There had never been a situation when I had allowed so much time to elapse before sharing a problem with him. We had always shared everything with each other. I had to give him the space now to go through his own paces before we could walk together on this. At this point, I had a three-month lead on this thought process. It hardly seemed fair. I was sorry that he knew, but I felt so relieved that he knew. I needed him. I couldn't do this on my own—I was too afraid to go it alone.

In the coming weeks, I obsessed a lot about losing my breast. I wondered how it would affect our relationship. I wondered how I would feel about myself, what it would do to my self-esteem. I had been feeling very troubled about an unusual amount of mid-life weight gain over the past five years and my self-esteem was running on low to empty, as it was. It had been a very long time since I felt that I was a desirable woman.

When my mother had her breast removed at age sixty, the thought of it sent me screaming right up the wall, at least inwardly. I had never been good about people being in pain, or having things cut off or cut into. Even watching a doctor give a needle on television caused me to turn away and wince. My mother was so brave about it all, and I was a complete mess. Is this how I would be now that it was my turn? I didn't want to think about it.

I struggled about when and what to tell the boys. Bruce became my compass. He guided me through that planning. When all my thinking was flying through the air like dandelion fluff, he helped me to come down to earth, to get centred and do what I had to do. We had a family meeting that night after dinner. My tone was matter-of-fact, but gentle. I made it a point to filter any fear from my voice. I told the boys that I would be going into the hospital in a few weeks—that there was a lump in my breast and that it was likely cancer. They were stunned. Their body language and facial expressions made a very brave attempt at normalcy. One got up and went silently into the bathroom. He didn't come back for a long while. The other asked flat out, "Will you have to have your breast removed?" "Most likely I will," I said, and quickly went on to point out that Grandma had had the same operation eighteen years ago and she was still tooting around at seventy-eight years of age. I saw some concern begin to lift, but only a little. Grandpa had died of cancer, they knew, and so had their uncle just a few years before. Cancer meant death. I could see it rushing into their thoughts. Mothers get to be mind readers after eighteen years of raising kids. At least we are pretty sure we can read minds. Sometimes, however, that can be delusional, I am told by family members— usually those whose minds I think I can read. Why wouldn't cancer mean death to my sons? It certainly did to Bruce and me.

There were a lot of quiet questions over the next few days. We were open with the boys about everything that we knew. A subtle and quiet sense of foreboding seemed to settle over our home. When one person in a family has cancer, the whole family has cancer. That's what it felt like. I could see the heavy burden begin to set in on all my men. It made me sad.

Bruce and I made a trip to the Cancer Society to pick up relevant booklets and to read them through, beginning to educate ourselves about this uninvited and surreal subject. I was hoping that the people at the Cancer Society would not be intrusive. I was not ready to talk to "outsiders" and I didn't want any well-meaning visitors to come to discuss my situation. To my relief, they were very respectful of this and very helpful. They didn't ask my name and I appreciated the anonymity. As we read the booklets, we shared the facts with the boys. As we learned, we began to wonder if there might just be a way to live through this trauma. One booklet stated that 50% of cancer patients go on to become survivors. That statistic held both good and bad implications depending on whether or not you viewed it from the "glass half full" or "glass half empty" perspective. I am usually the "half full" type myself but at this point, I was not operating in my usual mode. There was nothing very "usual" about any of this.

The next step was to tell my employer. I dreaded the outcome of that discussion. I anticipated losing my core employee job opportunity. This company was moving too far and too fast to have a sick person

in a key support position. My education told me that they couldn't
legally discriminate against me. The logic in that was clear but was a
small comfort. But what was important to me was to be hired as a
person of choice rather than as an obligation. My troubleshooting
instincts told me that I was not up to a legal battle, even if logic did
prevail.

The previously advertised formal job offer letter had not yet
arrived from my manager. It sounded as though this part of the
process could still be a month or so away, while yet another
restructuring study was finalized. The angst set in. Finally, I couldn't
stand it any longer. I wasn't about to sign an offer letter under false
pretenses and my nerves couldn't take another day of waiting to see if
my circumstances would be cause for concern. I phoned the leader of
our consulting team and laid it all out. The tension in my neck was
incredible. My heart was pounding. My mouth was dry.

I waited for the pause, the hesitation, the pronouncement that
this would need to be discussed with others and she would have to get
back to me. Legal would probably need to be consulted, the Wellness
Department would likely have an opinion and surely the vice president
of our department would have concerns about bringing me on board.
Just think of the family history, the implications if this person were to
cash in her chips within six months or even a year, they would say. Life
insurance would have to be paid and at what cost? What would the
company's liability be? People were being retired right, left and centre
to make way for the creation of a strong new company that would be
ready to meet the future.

As I finished the last detail of my unhappy story, my extrasensory
radar detected not a breath or hesitation. A steady, firm voice on the
other end of the line returned my communication by saying, "Get
yourself into surgery, get done whatever you have to do, and get back
to us when you can. Your job offer letter will be faxed to you and on
your desk tomorrow. You and your family will be covered by all the
benefits the company has to offer. I don't want you worrying about
these details at a time like this. Look after yourself, Pat, and let me
know if there is anything more that I can do for you."

I couldn't believe what I was hearing. My thoughts were running
rampant. Do you mean you will help me? Do you mean there is a

solution? Do you mean that I can relax and know that my family will be all right? Do you really, really mean that? Did I understand you correctly? Could you say it again? Could it be true? Could you say it again?

A million pounds of lead weight floated up from my shoulders and began to dissipate into thin air, before it even touched the ceiling. And true to my leader's word, the letter was on my desk the next morning. I could hardly wait to tell Bruce. A lifetime bond formed that day with the person who was my team leader. Whatever comes my way in life, no matter how old I grow to be, no matter what is in store for me after this life, I will never forget her kind and reassuring words and the fact that I was not an "obligation" but someone that she truly cared about.

Was a path beginning to form under my feet? In all the darkness and the impermeable fog, was there really a bridge up ahead that I might step onto to find my way? I had to be realistic. I didn't know if the path would take me to death or to further life; but just having a path to anywhere felt better than stepping out into oblivion.

Chapter **3**

Trolls Don't Just Live In The Forest!

A **week** after my appointment with the surgeon, I was to attend a
pre-admittance clinic at our local hospital—PAC, they called it.
Surgery was to be scheduled within two weeks or sooner. What kind
of surgery I was to have was unclear, but my guts were filled with
concern . . . I felt certain it would be radical.

I stepped into the PAC unit that morning feeling reserved and
rather quiet. I didn't want to be there. The PAC nurse greeted me and
began the process with recording my accurate weight. I thought I
detected her disapproval at the start, when I stepped on the scales and
she slid the balancing gizmo further and further down the line.
"THIS," she said, pointing to the number on her paper, "is what you
weigh." It felt like an accusation. "I'm quite aware of that," I thought
to myself, but nodded my head politely. I wasn't the least bit
impressed either, with my weight. We were in agreement there. It was
an awfully tender point and one that I didn't want jabbed or poked
today. I couldn't understand for the life of me why I had gained so
much weight in the past few years.

I followed her into the office. She proceeded to complete a
number of forms that would be helpful to the medical professionals
who would be working with me over the next while. There were a
myriad of questions about my health history, allergies, pregnancies,
medications, past surgeries, and so on. "Are you on a regular walking
program?" she asked. I replied that I was not. "Oh," she said, and
marked the questionnaire emphatically. That judgmental tension
seemed to form on her lips again, as she pursed them tightly together
and stiffened her spine into a most correct posture. I decided that I

wasn't imagining things. Her manner reminded me of the Church Lady I had seen so often on *Saturday Night Live*. Comedian Dana Carvey would say, "Hmmmm, let me see . . . could it be SATAN?" as he donned the puritan mode, hair tightly pulled back in a bun, and looked down from a pedestal through "her" horn-rimmed glasses in judgment of anyone "she" could get her beady little eyes on.

At that point in the interview, the nurse decided to take my blood pressure. As she attempted to attach the pressure cuff to my arm, she clucked away about having to go next door to get the LARGER size cuff. I was furious. I suspected that she knew the cuff wouldn't fit me before she even tried it. "It was probably a pressure cuff for children," I thought. "This woman should be shot." I knew that I had become overweight, but this dame was starting to make me feel like the fat lady in the circus, and logic told me that fifty new pounds did not put me in that category. It definitely put me on the wrong side of healthy, however, and I knew it. I didn't need to be told. "Never mind," I told myself, "someone made a real mistake staffing her in this position!" I thought about giving her an impromptu performance appraisal, but I couldn't muster the gumption to give her my feedback (right between the eyes). I sat there politely and quietly, while she retrieved the LARGER pressure cuff and I swallowed the humiliation.

The teaching portion of the process began. The Troll (as I had deemed her) gave me two articles to read—one on yellow paper about a lumpectomy and one on blue paper about a mastectomy. I glanced over the articles, noted the sections regarding what part of the breast would be cut and where. I began to feel nauseated and slightly dizzy. Her voice clipped out the points in perfect sequence, as she had apparently done 322 times earlier that week with other people. The rote nature of the exercise began to irritate me. She didn't seem to have any awareness of the gravity of my personal situation as it began to hit home in my heart. I was no longer listening to her words. Instead, I found myself watching her motions, marveling at how she could deliver the message in this manner. It seemed as though she was doing a cooking show on television about chicken livers, with no comprehension whatsoever of what this message meant to me, to my life.

When her words came back into focus she was lining up several cotton breasts from a big plastic bag of temporary prostheses and stating methodically, "Now, let me see. You are a very LARGE-breasted woman, so one like this might be appropriate for YOU!" as she smacked a great big cotton mound on the table in front of me. Is THIS what I was to make a trade for? My breast for this cotton-tail?

My eyes filled with tears and for a brief moment the Troll became compassionate. She offered me a tissue and some softer words of consolation. It might have crossed her mind how terribly sad this was. Regardless, she didn't know where the Cancer Society was, but suggested that I drop in to see them and pick up some reading material. How in the world could she be in charge of this exercise and not even know the address of the Cancer Society in a city of 65,000 people? A useless Troll at best, I thought!

I got up from my chair and walked quietly out the door. I didn't want to be there. I didn't want to be anywhere! I surely didn't want to be inside my own body. I felt a desperate need to reach up to my neck for the zipper of my flight suit, to pull it right down to my big toe, and to step out of my body, leaving it behind on the sidewalk. It was just a shell. Who needed it anyway? But I couldn't do that. I was trapped. Whom could I call? Whom could I negotiate with? My mind was darting into twenty places at once. There was no one. I was overwhelmed with the enormity of being soundly stuck with this situation, like it or not!

I found myself transposed into a crumpled leaf, floating through a swiftly moving current. I was heading quickly and without hope of rescue toward white-water rapids. There were no branches to grab, there was no ground below to touch with my feet, no rock ledge to wedge myself into, and no eagle above to pluck me safely out of the water. I had lost complete control of my body, my life and my future.

When I reached home and started telling Bruce about the whole dreadful experience, I burst into tears. He was outraged. Somehow that made me feel better. This was the first time I had completely lost my composure in front of anyone. "I don't want this!" I said over and over, stamping my foot. He put his arms around me and hugged me. There was nothing that could be done. "If you have to have a mastectomy," he said, "it is not going to make any difference as to how I feel about you. I'll love you whether you have three breasts or none." Those words meant so very much to me. I settled down and resigned myself to the fact that there was absolutely nothing on this agenda that was within my control.

In the months to come, I would learn a great deal about my feelings that day. I would think of a tool that I had used in my work with other people, but it was a tool that I had not thought to use for myself; not since the death of my daughter ten years before. I read in a wonderful book entitled *Return to Wholeness: Embracing Body, Mind and Spirit in the Face of Cancer* by David Simon M.D. (1999), that "the compassionate healer and researcher Elizabeth Kübler-Ross described five psychological stages that people go through when facing a life-threatening illness:

Denial, Anger, Bargaining, Depression and Acceptance."

At once I began to think about the healing cycle that I had used in a wonderful development program to help people through the loss caused by organizational change (Barger and Kirby 1997) (I have adapted the model to reflect my journey but the steps are essentially the same.)

This is a familiar psychological concept used to help people understand the steps involved in coping with personal losses such as death or divorce. Later, when I could be more objective, I would decide to adapt the "grieving cycle" to help me in understanding my own feelings in dealing with breast cancer and the journey that I was making. To this point, I had definitely been down the left side of the trough. In the months to come, I decided to rename this concept "the healing cycle."

My steps did not form a sequential path. They rarely do in such situations. I moved from one to the other, jumped ahead a bit, and fell back at times but continued to move through the cycle. Looking back on all that has transpired since then, I realize that there were many times when I had multiple cycles on the go over different issues at any point in time.

And immediately I could see my footsteps on the healing cycle during this Pre-Admittance Clinic. I never did change my mind,

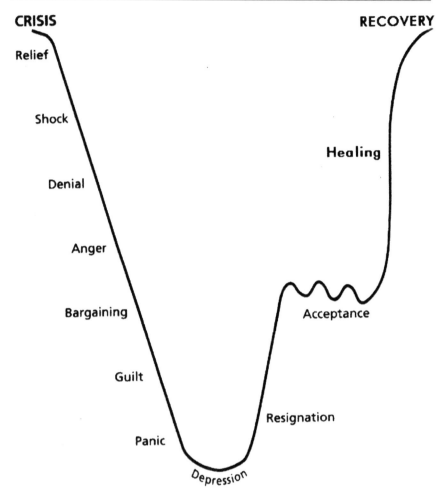

however, about the Troll. A Troll is a Troll by any definition. But I
also realized that this was the first time that **anger** had surfaced since
I awakened into this whole terrible mess. The PAC nurse was only a
person. I was willing to let it go. There were more important concerns
to move on with. It was gone but not forgotten.

Chapter 4

The Safety Net

Surgery was scheduled for the next morning. I was scrambling at work to get some loose ends tied up. I hadn't been planning on an absence. Multi-tasking had been my definite *modus operandi*, and as a result I had a lot of irons in the fire. A few of my close colleagues called to wish me well and provide their support. One of them had been through breast cancer surgery the year before. It was good to talk with someone who had lived the experience. I was most curious about what chemotherapy might be like. She gently described it as having a tiring impact, and for a few days after, like the worst flu she had ever had. But then it would pass and she would go in to work part time. There would be chemo nurses who would hook me up to an intravenous drip along with a lot of other patients. The IV itself would not be painful or uncomfortable. Everyone in the chemo unit would chat and before I knew it, the process would be over. It would take a few hours, she said. Hearing the step-by-step description from someone that I knew was helpful. It sounded livable.

There was work to hand off to others—not my customary mode, but nonetheless necessary. I hated piling work and responsibility on other people. Everyone seemed to be so busy as it was. Stress levels were building because of the ongoing organizational restructuring. Things were in chaos and people seemed to have slipped into the catacombs of the living dead, as they tried to put on a brave face to meet the challenges of the day, not knowing what the future was to bring for their careers. I alleviated my guilt by telling myself that I had a good excuse. After all, I had cancer.

The day ended. I locked up my filing cabinet, put my phone on "call forward," took a look around my office, and was satisfied that all was in order for the next few weeks. Then I'd be back and could pick up where I had left off. There was a lot to do when I returned, but people would just have to be patient until I got this "thing" out of my way. I packed a lot of work into my oversize briefcase. I could do some "catch-up" reading while I was off and perhaps get some plans in order that would speed up my efficiency level when I got back. I thought about taking my laptop computer home, but knew that would never pass Bruce's inspection when he arrived to collect me at five p.m. He would disapprove. I thought about all the times he had suggested that I leave my cell phone and computer at work when I came home for the weekend. "Give yourself a break," he would say. "You're working too much; you're going to burn out." Sometimes I would sneak things home and wait until he was out golfing. I just needed to preview a video, or read an article that I would have to present on Monday morning, or develop a new training program. It was the only opportunity that I seemed to get to do some creative work. Life at the office was non-stop phone calls and people needing to talk; emails seemed to propagate with every breathing moment and issue management was the order of the day.

My briefcase was packed. Only a few of the managers with whom I worked were aware that I was going to be away because of surgery for breast cancer. I said good night as usual to the rest of the staff and walked out the door. "I'll be back in about two weeks," I thought to myself. I'll take it slow and easy and everything will be just fine. I pressed the button for the down elevator without realizing that the cloak of denial was slipping itself around my shoulders once more.

Things were quiet at home that evening. We had dinner, watched television, took the dog out, all the usual activities, but it was not the same for anyone. There were no discussions. Each of the boys had come to me separately, in their own time, to talk. The initial question with both was to ask, "Mom, do you think there is any chance that you could die?" I had responded, "Not if I have any say in the matter!" I couldn't honestly deny the possibility, but it seemed to help them when they sensed that I still had some power over the situation.

It had helped so much in these discussions to remind them of Grandma's great success in her battle with cancer, which had occurred when they were only about a year old. It gave them perspective, I think, to consider that they were now nineteen and Grandma was still okay. It gave me perspective as well. I had read in the newspaper that of those women diagnosed with breast cancer this year, about two-thirds of the group would go on to become survivors. Not the best odds, I thought, but it was something to work with.

I went to sleep as soon as my head hit the pillow. It had been a big day. The next morning I was awake at four a.m. "Today is the day—the day that my life will change forever," I thought. In a few short hours, my left breast would be gone. I felt certain it was going to happen and shed a few quiet tears. I felt Bruce's arm gently surround me and knew that he was thinking the same thing. We fell back to sleep.

There were two notes on the kitchen counter that morning. They had been written the night before. One son had written *"Good luck with your surgery tomorrow Mom. Looking forward to seeing you again."* He was a man of few words. I knew him better than he realized. There were all sorts of messages and feelings behind those two short lines written on a yellow post-it note. He had told me of his worries that I might die like Grandpa. I knew that his quiet manner was concealing a lot of pain. Next to this, there was another handwritten note, from my other son:

> *"I said a prayer for you today, I know God must have heard;*
> *I felt the answer in my heart, although he spoke no word.*
> *I didn't ask for wealth or fame—I knew you wouldn't mind.*
> *I asked that he would send you blessings of a far more greater kind.*
> *I asked that he'd be with you—in all things GREAT and small!*
> *But, it was for his loving care I prayed for most of all.*
> *I love you Mom."*

My twins have very different personalities and communication styles, and yet I knew they would share equally in the stress and worry today. I remembered very well the thoughts that had gone through my own mind when my mother had her surgery. It had seemed so unfair, that such a harsh and cruel thing could be done to such a lovely, tiny person. That person had read *Winnie-the-Pooh* endlessly to me, and had made the most intricate little doll clothes and loved me so much through all my ups and downs as I grew through the years. And there had been a number of "downs." I was sorry that my sons had to experience this sadness. But I was also beginning to realize, regrettably, that I couldn't shield them from life.

My surgery was scheduled very early. Bruce and I were gone before the boys woke up.

We seemed to wait endlessly as we worked our way through the intake process at the hospital. I was very uptight. We did not converse much. Finally it was time to go. The porter was there with her gurney ready to wheel me off to surgery. Bruce walked with us. She seemed a no-nonsense sort as she manoeuvred her way through people and elevator doors that didn't want to wait for us. We seemed to go down, down to the basement of the hospital.

When we got off the elevator, she turned to my husband and officially said, "This is as far as you can go," and gave him directions to the "quiet room." He was to wait there to speak with the surgeon once the operation was finished. I could sense the muscles in his throat choke up as he kissed me and said, "take care." It felt as though we were saying goodbye to each other. The porter was obviously touched by the emotion between us. She wheeled me away to a hallway outside of the operating room, and patted my arm saying, "Don't worry, dear, you're going to be just fine. You've got the best surgeon going," and she left my side. "Oh good," I thought. "That's really good to hear—the best surgeon going!"

Half an hour seemed to pass. Doctors and nurses were passing by. I lay there quietly, reflecting on the situation. I realized that I was beginning to feel very calm for some reason. It was a peaceful feeling. Something was telling me that I didn't need to be afraid. And I wasn't. I thought about my mother and how she had blazed a trail for me. She was all right. I thought about the way that things were falling into place with my employment, the sick leave benefits that I needed so badly, and the support that everyone was giving to me. I reached a state of complete calm. I decided it was all going to work out for the best. What an unusual sense of peace, I thought. I wonder what has happened to make me feel this way? I smiled to myself. I knew the answer.

In a few moments, the surgeon came out to talk with me. She was very reassuring. I was brought into the operating room. The anesthetist began to do her work, all the while asking me about my children and engaging me in whatever chatty conversation she could think of. She was having trouble finding a good vein in my hand for the anesthetic. This had happened before on numerous occasions and was becoming a phobia of mine. It happened every time I needed an IV or a blood test, and I usually ended up being poked until I thought I would pass out. Elusive veins—what a plight! I usually managed to be polite and brave as long as I didn't watch. It was not particularly painful, but I did not cope well with having my skin pierced. A couple of attempts failed but my sense of calm did not leave me. The room was cool. I was glad of that.

The surgeon began to move my left breast in all sorts of different directions—only a talent that "large-breasted women" can have, I thought, mentally thumbing my nose at the Troll, who was somewhere three floors above us. The doctor began to draw things on my breast with a pen (directions, no doubt). I could tell from the manipulations that she was charting out a course to remove my breast and ensure that what was left would lie smoothly on my chest. For a brief moment, my heart sank. Whatever slight thoughts of a mere lumpectomy that might still have been lurking in the corners of my mind were now banished. The surgeon knew that it would be a mastectomy and now so did I, with complete certainty. All right then, I thought. I have faith that you will do a good job. And I silently gave her my permission to go ahead. The anesthetist had completed her mission, and I was gone, with no sensation of slipping away.

I don't remember much about waking up. I was in a hospital room with cheery draperies. The sun was coming through, lighting up soft pastels of pink and blue. My kindred spirit was there by my side, talking to me in his soft-spoken, gentle voice. I knew that my breast was gone without checking. There was no shocking moment to adjust to. I felt joyful at waking up and realizing that the deed was done and I had lived to tell the tale. I was not in any pain.

My spouse's second visit, that day, brought news from home. He had gone to connect with the boys and had explained the outcome of my surgery. He knew they would be waiting anxiously. I asked how they had received the news. My husband indicated that they had decided to clean the house from stem to stern and were busy vacuuming when he left. "Oh, that bad, huh?" I said. He smiled. We knew they were trying to find their own way to be supportive to us both.

I was to stay in the hospital overnight and go home the next day. I thought that was pretty neat. I had never enjoyed being in the hospital for very long—too boring. They were not trying to accommodate *me*, however. Rather, this was the new approach to keeping costs down, we speculated, and was permissible as long as the patient had someone at home to help care for her. Community Care would arrange to have the Victorian Order of Nurses come in every day to check on me. I was cheered by the thought of "getting out" the next morning.

My sons, my husband's beautiful daughter (and now mine), and her husband came in to visit that evening. I could see the stress written in every pore of their anxious faces. They were feeling my pain and I wanted so much to tell them that I really was not uncomfortable. I was all fixed up with Morphine, or Demerol, or something, and it was working very efficiently.

I was very touched by their depth of concern and caring. I had such an urge to wipe the slate clean for them, to take this depressing thing off the agenda, but I had lost my fairy godmother wand somewhere and here we all were. I was glad they had each other to share thoughts and concerns with, once they left. They seemed to want to keep things upbeat with me, in case I was depressed. The awkward gaps in our conversation were making them uncomfortable. I wasn't much help on that score; I was feeling a little pooped. They'd be okay, I thought.

The next morning my surgeon came in to see me. "Well, that was definitely cancer," she said, getting straight to the point. I liked that about her. "I am quite certain that there is lymph node involvement," she added, and asked me to come to see her in about ten days when the pathology report would be ready. We would talk then about next steps. She reminded me again that I would need chemotherapy because of my "young age." She added that I might need radiation as well. None of this was a surprise to me. My body had told me what I was up against. I was not confused about the state of affairs. My body had always notified me when I was pregnant, long before the medical tests confirmed it. I knew enough to trust it to announce any major changes, at least when I was using my internal "listening skills."

Very shortly after that, I was at home with a good supply of pain medication—just in case. It was wonderful to be home. My husband had prepared our bed with the cheeriest set of sheets. It was a few weeks before Easter and I remember thinking our queen-size bed looked like a giant Easter egg, with its pastel yellow sheets and mauve down comforter. The sunshine was coming in the window. It looked so inviting. I lay my head down and drifted off to sleep.

Every now and then Woody would drift through the room, checking on me. The nostrils of his nose would actively seek out the latest diagnostics, and he would stop long enough to be petted. He knew enough not to bump the bed. Under normal circumstances, Woody's sheep-herding instincts would cause him to bump emphatically up against the sides of the bed and then the foot of the bed in an attempt to get us up and at 'em. His ninety pounds could give the bed quite a series of jolts, when he wanted to. But his instinctual discretion prevailed.

The boys came in after school, full of news and relieved to see me home. And my soulmate would check on me often and sit for a while to talk. The VON nurses came and went each day, taking my temperature and my blood pressure. There were tubes in my side that had to be emptied of fluid. I made a point not to look at the tubes and was glad when enough time had passed and they were taken out. This was determined by the natural reduction in the amount of fluid that was present as each day passed.

It was so good to be home and to have that surgery behind me.

I had left strict instructions with my friends at work and in my personal life, that I did not want company. I much preferred to have everyone know me with my lipstick and high heels on. They respected that, but my goodness, they sent lovely flowers and cards and they phoned to see how I was. It was heartwarming! I had no idea that so many people would take the time to let me know they cared. The bouquets of flowers seemed to arrive every day for weeks, always a delightful interruption to our day.

On the fifth day after my surgery, I went through a sad spell. It had taken me that long to muster the nerve to take a look at my incision. Until then, I had managed to change my pajama top while looking out the bedroom window, or at my foot, or anywhere else that seemed a pleasant diversion. But today I decided it was time to take a look. It was as I had imagined—very neatly done. That side of my chest reminded me of many years ago, when I was a little girl with no breasts. I went back to bed and began to think about the day that my mother and I had purchased my first bra at the local department store. I was eleven years old; the bra was a 28 AA. It was merely a Band-Aid, but I was extremely proud of it. I was filled with a deep sadness at losing this part of my body, an old friend that had represented so much of my womanhood.

When the nurse arrived that day, she cheerily asked my husband the usual, "So—how's it going?" He advised her that I might be feeling a little down. Without comment, she slipped up the stairs to our bedroom, wrapped her arms around me and said, "It's okay to cry, you know." That unleashed a huge flow of emotion. It reminded me of when I was a child and would fall and scrape my knee on the way home from school. I would walk the rest of the way home with my friends without crying. Acting like a baby was out of the question. Then I would get in the door and my mother would say, "What happened to your knee?" and a whole flood of tears would rush forth while she hugged me and I told her all about the terrible incident. I am so grateful to that nurse for her professionalism and empathy. She had all the right timing, the right listening skills and the right words.

I cried most of the afternoon and then the sadness passed.

I settled into a huge safety net that was laid out carefully for me by my family. I rested in bed and treasured the delicious opportunity not to be busy. My mind was full of deep thoughts. The oversized briefcase, stuffed with undone work, was millions of miles from my thinking. It lay gathering dust in the basement. At times, I would decide that I wanted to go downstairs to the living room to watch television with everyone. My husband provided the escort down a double set of staircases and would just get me nicely settled on the sofa when I would announce that I thought I was tired and would have to go back up to bed. The long journey would put me nicely back to sleep.

After two weeks of resting at home, I began to worry about returning to work. I didn't feel up to it. I confided my concerns with the VON nurse one afternoon. She was shocked that I could even consider returning to work after only two weeks. She firmly emphasized that I had had major surgery and would not be able to think about returning to work for at least six to eight weeks. I was secretly so relieved. I just didn't have the energy. I settled back on my pillow and let all the tension leave my body. All seemed to be quite well. I was just so tired. A little more time to rest was just what I needed.

The first day that I got up and dressed was the day I went for my follow-up appointment with the surgeon. I was filled with anticipation, knowing that the surgical pathology report would be ready to discuss. I was expecting a verdict of "lymph node involvement." Sure enough, we got right to the point, and that was the point. The surgeon explained that this meant I was "already at Stage 2 cancer." I didn't know what that meant, but would learn about it. I asked with an expressionless face, "So when do you think I can go back to work?" She thought for a minute, looking at the ceiling, calculating the treatment that she knew would be needed and then responded, "It will be at least four to five months to go through the chemotherapy program and you may need radiation after that." The words slammed into me. I almost physically fell off the examining table. Five months! What were they thinking? I couldn't be off work for five months! Did she perhaps mean five *weeks*? "Okay," I said quietly, still no expression. She eyed my face very carefully and walked over to her file to make some notations. I felt uncomfortable about being read so easily. She seemed to know that it wasn't okay with me at all, despite my controlled reaction.

As I was getting my shoes on, the surgeon handed me a written copy of the pathology report. "This is for your records," she said. I was delighted. I had never had the privilege to be given my own medical facts in writing before—and I could take them home with me. I felt very empowered. I needed time to read the report over, to study it and understand it. I might have questions. I wanted Bruce to read it.

The surgeon noted that she would want me to go for some tests in a few weeks: a liver scan and a bone scan. Geeeeeez! I thought. Is there going to be more? Then she explained that this would provide a baseline they could compare with in the months to come. "A likely story," I thought. I assumed she suspected there were more problems and this was a gentle way of easing me into the test without causing added worry. And then she added, "There was an abnormality on the ultrasound of your liver, so we'd like to check that out." She wrote out a medical slip for my employer. It said, *"This woman will need to be off work for the next 4 to 5 months."*

I found my husband in the waiting room. I was speechless, winded with the magnitude of the situation. We walked to the car and along the way he asked me as casually as he could, "So, how did it go?" The words wouldn't come. I handed the medical slip over to him. He was as shocked as I had been. We drove home without much discussion. The report had a lot of information that we were not yet equipped to understand. But the highlights stood out, nonetheless.

The more significant sections read as follows:

MICROSCOPIC DESCRIPTION:

QUICK SECTION MICRO:

The section is hypercellular and consists of pleomorphic malignant cells showing rare lumen formation. The malignancy extends to the inked margin.

Specimen A: [the lump] *Sections reveal a high grade invasive malignancy that is permeating the breast stroma and fat. It is composed of large epithelioid malignant cells showing a high degree of nuclear pleomorphism and having large irregular eosinophilic nuclei. Mitotic activity is brisk, upwards of 35 mitosis per 10 high power fields are counted. The malignant cells are arranged in irregular nests as well as solid sheets. They show areas of central necrosis reminiscent of* *comedocarcinoma. Lumen formation is identified as greater than 10% of the tumour consistent with an SBR score of 2/3 for lumen formation. The marked nuclear pleomorphism and mitotic activity gives a total SBR score of 8/9. The malignancy extends to within 0.1 mm of the nearest inked margin. There is a moderate inflammatory reaction to the infiltrating tumour with a rim of lymphocytes and plasma cells at the advancing borders. There are some areas that are highly suspicious for vascular invasion.*

Specimen B: [the balance of my breast] *The nipple displays no evidence of Paget's disease. Dermal lymphatics do not contain any metastatic tumour nests. The hematoma margin contains benign breast lobules and ducts. The deep surgical margin is free of malignancy. Random sections of breast tissue reveal benign lobules and ducts. There is a mild degree of fibrocystic change. Six auxiliary lymph nodes are identified. All show metastatic tumour.*
5 of 6 lymph nodes have been almost completely replaced by the metastatic tumour.

Final diagnosis:
Specimen A: Left breast (biopsy)
  infiltrating poorly differentiated ductal carcinoma
  A) SBR Score 8/9
  B) Suspicious for vascular invasion
  C) Extension within 0.1 mm of nearest excisional margin

Specimen B: Left breast (complete mastectomy and auxiliary dissection)
  – no residual malignancy identified
  – 6/6 auxiliary lymph nodes positive for metastatic tumour
  – excision margins free of malignancy

There was a lot to absorb, in spite of previous notification from my body. Understanding this information on an emotional and intellectual level required some heavy-duty thinking. I felt numb. My thoughts were overwhelmed with detail. I couldn't deal with all this right now . . .

I suddenly realized that I had better think about getting my tax return completed. The due date was only a few weeks off. Of course, I could die and that would fix "their" wagons! I was angry that I had to do my tax return at a time like this. "Cancer patients should be excluded from that damned yearly ritual," I thought. How dare they, the crass, insensitive money grabbers! I grumbled around about tax laws for the rest of the day, gathering receipts and digging out my records. It seemed milder fodder than thinking about my lymph nodes busily transporting cancer cells to every corner of my body. Besides, I needed to get everything in order; just in case, my subconscious was saying—just in case.

Chapter 5

The Tunnel

I felt as though I was stepping into a long tunnel. I visualized myself alone inside the tunnel. I could see my husband walking beside me along the outside of the wall. Anytime I put my hand on the surface of the tunnel, Bruce would put his palm against mine, so I didn't feel completely alone. Inside the tunnel it was very dark and at some point it seemed to angle upward, forcing me to climb and climb. I was sure that I could see a glimmer of light miles ahead. This sense of light gave me great hope. "This is a long journey that I have to make," I told myself. "But in the end, I will get to that light and everything will be all right." I instinctively knew there would be significant challenges along the way, but I also felt sure that I could meet them head on. I had a strong feeling of conviction on that score. When I told my husband about the tunnel, he listened intently; his facial expression told me that the hair on the back of his neck was standing straight up.

One of the managers with whom I work is known for a particular comment that he makes when all hell is breaking loose. After an intense team meeting, he'll stand fully erect, and in his casual deep voice, he will drawl, "Well boys, I think we're seeing a light at the end of the tunnel here—I just hope to hell it isn't a train!" And everyone will laugh and shake off the tension of the moment. I thought about that in connection with my tunnel and smiled.

We were very busy the next few weeks going to appointments at the hospital for blood tests, liver scans and bone scans. The anticipation of the results of those tests was hard to take at times. My father had colon cancer that had spread significantly to his liver and he died in six short months. My aunt died of breast cancer years before. It had spread to her bones and had given her a very difficult time. "Of course, that was at least twenty years ago," I reminded myself. But while waiting for the verdict on the rest of my organs for the next few weeks, it was difficult to keep my imagination in check.

I was in touch with my regional director (my business partner) off and on through email from my home computer—sometimes checking in on business, other times letting him know how I was doing. Both his mother and father had gone through cancer as well. We shared that history. These were discussions about our personal lives that we had not had before. He asked one day over the "air waves" what the prognosis was for my case. I responded on my keyboard that I had read that 50% of cancer patients go on to be survivors, so my assumption was that my own chances were 50/50. His response to me was one of the best pieces of advice I received throughout this experience and I never let go of it. Here is what he wrote to me:

> "On cancer, it seems to me that there are more experts than answers. My thoughts are that you should know all there is to know from a factual perspective, i.e., what it is, how it works, what causes it to occur, what kinds there are (know thine enemy). Statistics don't seem to me to be of much real value. My mom's chances [colon cancer] were first of all 20/80 (great depression), then 40/60 (40% looks good after 20, some hope arises) then six months of chemo; and she is living, breathing proof of how big statistics can beat you up when you're down or convince you of things that aren't true when you are up. Seems to me that it is you, at this very instant, that needs the attention, not obscure mathematical principles few understand and even fewer care to."

I stopped thinking about the 50/50 proposition. And later on, when I had the opportunity, I didn't even ask, "So what are my chances?" I decided to make a firm assumption that they were good! At times, I wondered if this was another of my indirect denial tricks. But through a discovery that was totally new to me, the principles of *mind/body medicine*, I learned that I had taken the right approach.

I like to "people-watch," and this entertained me while we waited for appointments at the hospital. One day we sat waiting for tests in Nuclear Medicine, which was located in the very bowels of the hospital. I was thinking about how depressing it must be to come to a dungeon to work every day. We patients sat waiting, full of some odd fluid that we had been asked to drink. Many were comparing health notes, which really didn't appeal to me. The magazines were literally over ten years old—collectors' items, at best. My husband was amused by issues of *Good Housekeeping* and *Better Homes and Gardens* dating as far back as 1989. We wondered if this was a subliminal complaint from the hospital regarding the severe budget cuts to health care.

As I entertained myself watching people coming and going, I began to notice how many breast cancer "ladies-in-waiting" were there. I zeroed in because every one of them was coming to the hospital with a dip in her chest—like a shallow bunker on the 9th hole—a tell-tale sign. I had put on a comfy, giant loose sweatshirt that morning, and there was that bunker in my chest, just like the procession I was watching. I had not cared until now. What the heck, I thought—my shirt was a delicious honeydew melon colour and it was clean. But after watching a reflection of my chest walking by on every second female, now it mattered. I was not in a state of grief over the situation, but rather becoming conscious of the fact that I would have to do some thinking about how to get around this fashion challenge so that I didn't look depressing to my family and to others. There seemed no need for everyone else to experience my wound to that degree. But it was too soon after surgery to be professionally fitted with a prosthesis.

We had been invited for Easter dinner to our daughter and son-in-law's home. Normally, when we gathered together, we were a troup of four adults, two six-foot teenagers, three spaniels and one giant Woody dog. It was a nostalgic family atmosphere at their home on the lake. I wanted it to be a happy and fun occasion for everyone.

I called the Cancer Society. It seemed like a good time to collect that "cotton tail" that I had been so indignant about. I would need the temporary prosthesis to get by for now. I wanted to get all fixed up for the holiday. But they were all out of stock and expecting an order sometime soon. I was miffed. How could the Cancer Society run out of breasts, for heaven's sake!

I was determined not to accept defeat. I took the shoulder pads out of a few dresses and stuffed them into the vacancy in my bra. It wasn't easy achieving balance with my right breast, my buddy, who had managed to survive the storm. Begrudgingly, I looked for four more shoulder pads to up the ante. Okay, so maybe I am a *fairly* large-breasted woman! It worked. I marched off to show my husband my new creation. He was mighty impressed. We had a good giggle together. The Easter dinner celebration was great and not one person in my family looked sad or worried when they talked to me. It was a "Good Thing."

Lynda called, Deb called, Darlene called, Sandra called, Karen called, Betty called, and my mother called and sent cards for weeks on end. These were all people with whom I had shared special "life moments." My aunts and my cousins and friends of my mother's sent continuous wishes of support and prayers for my well being. There was so much caring and support offered by so many people.

Through all of this, one thing completely captured my attention. It was a beautiful card from Lynda with a note inscribed inside. She told me of a book that she had read by a Canadian author, Penelope Williams (1993). The book was called *That Other Place: A Personal Account of Breast Cancer*. It was the story of the author's journey through breast cancer, and Lynda noted that she had been quite caught up in it. I knew that Lynda was an avid reader, but I found it unusual that she would read about breast cancer. Disease had certainly never been on my own reading list. I puzzled about whether she had gone through the experience herself and not shared it with me. She listed the library tracking number and recommended it as something that I "might want to read." For some reason, Lynda's note created a sense of urgency in me that I found difficult to understand; but I knew that I must follow through on it.

There was something unique about our friendship. I remembered her casual phone call a few years before, when she had a job ad to recommend to me, with a notion that there was a slight chance that I might be interested. It was a long shot, considering the proposition that I would leave an eleven-year career, a good pension and all the trappings for a one-year contract in an entirely different business. But Lynda knew that I was unhappy in my job and that I couldn't grow anymore, and she just had a feeling this might be good to mention. As it turned out, I walked away from my unhappy job, left all the security behind me, and went on to this opportunity as free as a butterfly and relieved to have escaped the "golden handcuffs." It was one of those experiences where you step back and take a second look at a friend and wonder if she is a guardian angel in disguise. And now it seemed to be happening again.

Lynda had gone to the trouble of sourcing the library tracking number for this book. To me that meant that I had to get that book, and I had to get it immediately. There was a reason. I didn't know what it was, but I knew it would unfold when the time was right. Within ten minutes of returning from the library I was reading the introduction and was in tears—and I don't cry easily. The author was already dedicating her words to the people with whom she had come into contact. Some had survived, some had not.

My husband looked worried. I could tell he was wondering if this was wise.

I read and I read and I read. So many of the author's thoughts and feelings were similar to my own. I was filled with anticipation as I read through the pages. I could tell that the book was very factual, and that it would shed light for me on the unknown nature of what I was to experience in the months ahead. I didn't want to know, but the suspense was driving me crazy.

A few chapters into the book, the author wrote about feeling that she was inside a long, dark tunnel. Geeeeeeeez! I almost threw the book across the room, fearful that it might be alive and was somehow reading my thoughts. How could she be writing about the tunnel? And then I realized that many, many people must have walked inside that tunnel before me, and that many had yet to find their way. It stopped me in my tracks. I thought that over in significant depth. It was like visiting an historic location, like the Great Wall of China, and feeling a bond, a linkage with mankind, knowing that so many people in the world had paid homage to that great location for centuries past and stood on the very spot that I was standing. I was awed.

I was exhausted when I crawled into bed that night. There were so many thoughts going through my mind. I dreamed and dreamed. Somewhere early on in my dream journey, the tunnel lost its definition. I found myself coming out into the dark night of an open field. The moon was shining above to provide at least some light on the situation. I could see a dense forest very far ahead in the distance, and mountains beyond that. The field was massive. All was silent. I didn't know which way to go. I called out into the night and heard my voice echoing back, "Can anyone tell me where the path is?" There was no answer. "I have to get on with my journey," I called out. "Please tell me where the path is." There was only silence as the soft wind touched my cheeks and sent a shiver through my body. I felt very alone. The connection that I felt earlier that day with all the others who had walked before me was gone. They were not answering me. Why wouldn't they help? I awoke at three a.m. feeling very troubled. I went quietly downstairs, made some peanut butter toast (a good cure-all), and picked the book up again.

As I read on, I could see that there were differences in our journeys. I was not feeling as bitter and angry as the author. There were differences in the medical treatment, partly because of the point in time that this author was being treated and, of course, because of the specifics of our individual breast cancer. And there were differences in the way we responded to our challenges, this author and I. Regardless of what was different or similar, it was through this reading that I was introduced to the field of mind/body medicine and the knowledge that this could help me to find my way through this terrible experience. The author connected me to the work of Deepak Chopra, *Quantum Healing—Exploring the Frontiers of Mind/Body Medicine* (1989) and *Ageless Body, Timeless Mind* (1993), and to the work of Dr. Bernie Siegel, *Love, Medicine and Miracles* (on audiotape or in book format), and so much more. I was so grateful to her for putting these clues on paper for me like crumbs leading through the forest. I had certainly heard of these authors before, but had never had an interest or a belief in learning about healing.

I read that chemotherapy would create havoc with my immune system, causing my white and red blood counts to deteriorate with each chemo session. Chemotherapy apparently doesn't distinguish between good cells and bad cells. I knew that a weakened immune system could open the door for other cancers to develop. I envisioned my cancer-invaded lymphatic system as an efficient transportation system—my internet, a super-highway, moving quickly throughout my body. It worried me. My blood counts would restore themselves, I learned, but I knew that I would need to have my immune system as a very strong ally.

Dr. Chopra (1989) wrote,

> "It is absolutely normal to be too busy to be sick, for that is exactly the kind of awareness that the immune system thrives on. When you are just yourself and not a "cancer patient," then the complicated chain of the immune response, with its hundreds of precisely timed operations, goes to work with a vengeance. But once you give in to helplessness and fear, this chain breaks apart. You start sending out the neuropeptides associated with negative emotions, these latch onto the immune cells, and the immune response loses its efficiency. (Exactly how this happens is not known, but the decreased immune status of depressed patients is well documented.) Here is where the paradox comes in: if you reacted to cancer as no great threat, the way you react to the flu, you would have the best chance of recovering, yet a diagnosis of cancer makes every patient feel totally abnormal. The diagnosis itself sets up the vicious cycle, like a snake biting its tail until there is no more snake" (p. 250).

Once I realized the significant power I held to shape my own healing, the feelings of helpless abandon began to leave me. I was beginning to realize that I could be an active participant in getting well. There was much to learn. I was on a high.

As I read through *Quantum Healing*, I wrote at the top of a page, *"Be a participant in the treatment; don't participate in the disease."* The message was coming through loud and clear. It became my mission. I knew I was on to something. I began to fervently research the tools that would help, and they were all tools that I could use inside my own mind. This was a concept with which I was comfortable. It took me back to being in charge of my own destiny.

I was becoming an architect, a mason, a builder of a pathway—the stepping stones that would lead up the mountain of my journey. I deeply understood the silence that I had experienced in the open field the night before. I was going to have to find my own way, not someone else's. There didn't seem to be any point in stopping to ask for directions. There would be familiar landmarks along the way that others had experienced, but for my own journey, it seemed evident, the path would have to be of my own creation.

Chapter 6

Mind Over Matter

Looking back, I can see that I didn't disconnect completely from work until I had been away from it for a full two months. At first, even though my body was at rest (at least figuratively speaking), my mind churned onward with the plans and issues of my workplace. It wasn't worry but rather a need for my brain to be planning, designing, creating, producing, accomplishing. One afternoon as I was resting in bed enjoying the sun streaming in the window, the realization came over me that I was beginning to disconnect from work. I had not been consciously aware that I was still plugged in. The constant chatter of thoughts rushing through my mind was enough to keep anyone preoccupied. The busyness of all that flurry had been quite stressful. I felt my body begin to relax, reminding myself again that I wasn't responsible for anything except getting better. It felt delicious. I marveled at the notion that the usual two-to-three-week vacation period from work was supposed to bring one renewal. At this point in my life, it wouldn't have even taken the seal off the cap. This challenge of balancing work and life was something I would have to think more about.

It was difficult to retain that feeling of peace. In the absence of puzzles to solve from work, I found my interest turning to world issues on CNN. I turned the television on each morning to check on the "breaking news." These days, there were not many dull moments. The Serbs and Kosovars were in a major internal struggle in Yugoslavia. I found myself intrigued with the daily reports of the bombing from the top brass at NATO and fascinated with learning the history of the strife in this country. Over the next few weeks, my mind began to strategize on the best approaches to resolve the issues in everyone's best interests. I watched as women and children and the very elderly climbed their way through the mountains, some transported in wheelbarrows, some in bare feet. The extreme hardship, rage and grief were tapping my greatest sense of empathy. Family members had been killed in the most horrendous of ways. I wondered how these people would ever heal and continue on with life, once all this was settled.

Then the shooting at Columbine High hit the airwaves. Memories of my daughter's life and death as a teenager swelled forth. We watched the whole incident transpire on the television screen and watched the aftermath for days afterward. I began to worry about the safety of my two sons at their own local high school.

I woke up one night with an audiotape playing on fast-forward through my mind. The narrative of the news and commercials that day was on loud volume, like a song that plays incessantly in your thoughts, until you get a headache from it. I got up and went into the bathroom. The reality of my surroundings were gently bringing me out of the war room and the mountains of Kosovo and back to my own safe North American haven. "I wasn't responsible for settling this war; this is completely outside of my circle of influence," I told myself. My life was not directly connected to what was happening at Columbine and my sons were perfectly well and safe. What on earth did I think I was doing, getting so caught up in all this?

I planned to spend the day with classical music playing and questioned why I couldn't just get used to having the room silent and enjoy the peace. It was confusing to know what to do with time, when one was not at work. It seemed that I was filling the absence of work in my mind with other issues. So many years at work, running around and around like a little hamster on a wheel, was going to be difficult to reprogram. If I didn't adjust it, someone would soon be saying, "The wheel's still turning, but the hamster's dead!" I had to know when to jump off. The time was now.

I would have to learn to relax and let my mind be empty, if that was at all possible. The more I thought about it, the more difficult a proposition that became. The next morning, I was on the Internet at my favourite bookstore. I often find my answers through reading. I remembered what Deepak Chopra had written about learning to live IN the moment. I constantly think in panoramic view, getting way ahead of myself, digging up countless options and ideas, planning towards the future. I would have to learn to focus on the absolute here and now. There is a saying: "Yesterday is gone and tomorrow isn't here yet, so what is there to worry about?" (Siegel, 1991) I would have to learn to get more in touch with my inner unconscious self, if I was to find the peace of mind that I knew was so crucial to my healing.

I ordered a set of books on tape by Dr. Bernie Siegel (1991). Unknowingly, I was opening the door to the learning and conditioning that was to help so much in the months ahead. The most helpful to me in this collection was *Love, Medicine, and Miracles*. While resting in the afternoon, I listened as Dr. Siegel talked to me about cancer and the patients he had known. He considered himself "The Privileged Listener," because of the opportunities he had had throughout his career as a surgeon to talk with both people who were dying and people who became survivors. I wanted to learn whatever techniques I could, to teach my mind to take on the unfathomable power of which I knew it was capable. I had a strong belief that if I could just get my mind re-educated in taking charge of my life in a more appropriate way, my body would respond in kind. I wanted this knowledge to help me through cancer and then to help me with my life, and with finding the balance that I so badly needed.

I learned about choosing the medical therapy that was right for me, a program that I personally could believe in. Dr. Siegel talked about nutrition and exercise, relaxation through meditation, guided imagery and visualization, and so much more. I had touched on these things in my life, but never delved all that deeply into them, because, of course, I was too busy.

Meditation and guided imagery were both techniques that appealed very strongly to me. It would help me to focus all that unchannelled mental chatter. I learned that I could greatly influence the side effects that I would experience through chemotherapy and radiation, by preparing my mind and my outlook in the most constructive way possible. Many people suffer from anticipatory nausea and other peripheral conditions due to their fear of the treatment and the imagined results. This is not to say that it's all in their heads, but I do believe that's where it starts—isn't that where everything begins? I would need to pull up those seeds before they could germinate.

I decided to use my strategizing energies to prepare for the challenge. I already understood the action of chemotherapy. I had read that it would kill cancer cells that were multiplying at mad random within my body. I also knew that the chemo could not distinguish between destructive rapidly dividing cancer cells and the good rapidly dividing cells in my body, like hair cells—and that this was the reason I would have to temporarily lose my hair. I had a preconceived notion that it was cancer that made people's hair fall out. Once I understood the rationale, I was okay with it. After all, if hair was falling out, the medicine was working and cancer cells were dying.

Dr. Siegel noted that many people are disturbed by destructive images of killing things within their own bodies. He recommended that visualizations be thought of in animated form with a positive twist—like white pussycats (white cells) eating cat food (cancer cells), thus creating a less destructive image.

I was able to come up with a visualization that connected to something I was familiar with in my profession—Conflict Resolution. I thought of my cancer cells as confused, misguided cells that were having trouble finding their way. Once again, Deepak Chopra (1989) educated me as follows: "*Cancer is a wild anti-social behaviour, whereby a single cell reproduces itself without check, heeding no signals from anywhere except, apparently, its own demented DNA. Why this occurs, no one knows. It is a good bet that the body itself knows how to reverse the process, but for some reason, equally unknown to science, it doesn't always succeed. It is only a matter of time, once the process begins, before the cancer cells overwhelm a vital organ, crowd out its normal cells, and cause death*" (p. 42).

I intended to have no part in that! I would transpose myself into a miniature facilitator and enter my body to help the good and the misguided cells to find harmony. Once the conflict had been fully discussed, the cancer cells would understand their new role and would willingly resume their original intelligence and stop multiplying or agree to move on, to be flushed from my system by chemotherapy. I thought of the chemo not as a toxic substance creating destruction within my body, but as a welcome miracle that would eliminate any toxins, bringing me renewal and a completely fresh start. There would be no conflict at all, only consensus decisions and a wiser understanding of what was needed by the cells in my overall system. The challenge would require my most masterful mediation skills.

I involved the people that I know from my workplace in my visualization. There were now tiny engineers manning the valves and engines of my internal systems. Al, Andrew, Gerry and Marcel were all there in their work boots, hard hats and safety glasses. It was crucial that they wear their safety equipment, so the cancer cells could not harm them. Richard is sitting at his drafting desk and the maintenance resource coordinators are just down the hall, ready to strategize the maintenance activities of all concerned. Elaborate schematics are consulted in order to most efficiently bring things to order. They were all there to support me in my conflict facilitation and would take over the controls if the going got tough.

Through my visualization, I learned to hold a cell in my hand. It is about the size of a pink party balloon. I move my hand across the outside of it but without touching and the cell begins to glow because I have the special power to do that. Once healed, I return it to its place of origin. The cell is relaxed and soothed.

These are not games that I play. I am activating my mind to influence physical systems within my body to effect changes that will actually take place. It is entirely possible to control one's heartbeat or to shrink tumours, through visualization. I know that I have the power to do this and I am euphoric over the anticipated outcome. I also know that there could be trouble along the way. But I am prepared to strategize those challenges. In *That Other Place,* by Penelope Williams (1993), there was a notion that stayed with me. Many cancer patients experience a recurrence, but it doesn't have to mean it is the end. She suggests that the challenge be thought of as a boxing match with a potential ten rounds. I would win some and I might lose some, but it was the overall match that really counted. I was ready and getting more and more ready every day. I was developing resilience and confidence, the survivor traits that would be needed.

Chapter 7

The Plan

We finally received the call to attend an appointment with an oncologist at our regional cancer centre. The date was to be almost six weeks from the date of my surgery. The stress had been building. That seemed like a long time to leave cancer unmonitored, sneaking around my body at will. And then we were still awaiting the results of my liver and bone scans. What a huge relief when the call finally came.

RELIEF. That brings my thoughts back to the healing cycle. By now, the trough on that cycle was beginning to look like the bowl of my food processor. And we had been inside with the button turned on, bouncing back and forth and up and down, through all the emotions and stages. RELIEF was right back at the beginning stage of the cycle.

"Now we'll get some answers," we thought. Now we'll hear what the treatment is to be. Now, we'll finally know what the score is! A big deep breath from both of us, and then a sigh of relief. Not knowing much of anything for a whole six weeks had been very tough. The "unknown" is so difficult to deal with; it is the root of all fear. Bruce and I were annoyed at times that the system wasn't getting me right in as a priority case, but we knew that the volume of cancer patients was unreal and we would just have to wait for an opening. Later, I understood there was also the concern of allowing my body some time to heal from my surgery, before starting chemo.

The cancer centre was about a two-hour drive from our home. We stocked up on coffee and muffins at the local drive-thru and made our way down the highway. It was a sunny, spring morning. We both

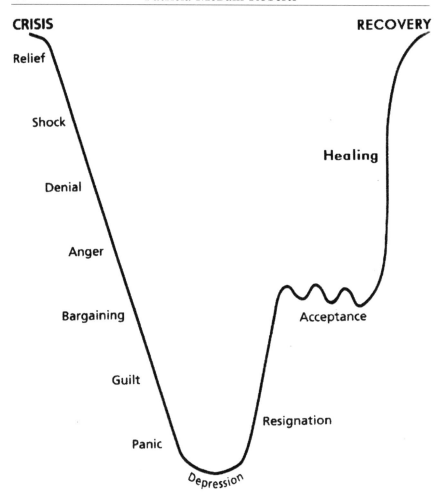

loved spring. We chatted all the way, enjoyed the scenery and the freshness of the season. It had been a long winter; a troubled winter.

On arrival, my husband and I were impressed with the architecture of the building we were entering. It appeared to be state-of-the-art . . . not at all like the bowels of the hospital we had been sitting in for tests the past few weeks. Inside, there was wonderful artwork, bright sunny skylights, and *comfortable* seating areas for patients in waiting. The latter struck us as a novel concept, to be sure. There were pods of volunteers, all in bright daffodil yellow coats—most appeared to be seniors. They were friendly folks, glad to be there, glad to be helping out. One volunteer welcomed us very warmly and asked if it was our first visit. With this confirmed, she took us under her wing and set about explaining the intake process and where to find everything, including the coffee and cookies that were in the waiting area. I was checked in by an administrative person, and was impressed with the personable and reassuring approach she took to the conversation. It seemed so different from the usual stressed hospital administration we had experienced at home.

We were early. I wandered around, reviewing small libraries of books encased in glass bookshelves. I loved books. They were all there to be borrowed by anyone who had a notion to read. There was everything from nutrition and medicine, to humour for cancer patients and their families.

When I finally took my place beside Bruce in the waiting area, I noticed that we had both become very quiet. He was engrossed in a pamphlet of information. I looked up at the ceiling and felt a flood of uncertainty rush over me. My mood was changing dramatically. The prior feelings of *relief* had left me completely. "What am I doing sitting here in a cancer center?" I thought. A *cancer centre*, for heaven's sake! Me? What has transpired in my life to bring me here? How could I have possibly developed cancer? This was real. . . . I was now officially becoming a "cancer patient." I looked around the waiting area at a few other early arrivals. They looked like quiet, sad people. The tears began to well up. I didn't want to be there anymore. I had waited six weeks to get there, was annoyed about the delay, and now I didn't want to be there. Fear has no logic. My husband sensed the upset and began to gently coach me through it. I settled to some degree.

My name was called and we both rose to follow the primary nurse to an examining room, where I was to meet my oncologist. The nurse was a friendly and assertive sort. Her conversation pulled me out of my thoughts and back to the moment. She handed me a hospital gown and asked me to prepare for an examination. "The doctor will be in in a minute," she said, "and he has a very long story to tell you." We waited in silence. When they came back in to see us together, I was immediately amused by the doctor's chocolate-brown bow tie, sprinkled with tiny yellow giraffes. I decided he must be quite human and I would keep him. There was little acknowledgement from either of them regarding my husband sitting in the corner of the examining room. I was concerned about that. All the pamphlets I had read, encouraged the patient to bring a spouse or a friend, so that they could help in hearing all the information that was to be communicated. As the doctor talked, I worried that Bruce was feeling left out. After all, we were in this together.

The nurse had not misled us. It seemed that the doctor talked for a very long time. In real time, it might have been ten or fifteen minutes. The facts of my own case were interwoven with facts about breast cancer and potential treatments. There was so much information. From what I recall, we learned that my bone scan had been fine. Phew! I had been sent for the wrong kind of liver scan and this would have to be redone at my local hospital. The ultrasound of my liver, however, had shown an abnormality that he felt was very important to identify. A vision of my father's face as he lay on his deathbed flashed through my mind.

And then, of course, there was the issue of six out of six of my lymph nodes having cancer "involvement." We knew this already. He asked when I had first discovered the lump. I was honest this time, and told him that it had actually been three to four months prior to my surgery. He appeared to be disturbed that I had not had more significant follow-up treatment when the "pre-cancerous" cells had been removed eight years earlier. I was watching his face carefully; my extrasensory perception was turned on high frequency to absorb any signals that might tell me if he thought I was going to die. Gazillions of thoughts were racing through my mind. At the same time I was trying to listen to his words.

I noticed that he deliberately steered away from any talk of statistics. I had learned in my research that talk of statistics was actually quite detrimental to cancer patients. It is the whole mind/body thing. Once a doctor (the voice of authority and wisdom) speaks of predicted statistical odds to a patient, it can become a very real influence in how the patient responds to healing. If patients are told they have six months to live, the impact of that statement can help the prediction to materialize. On the other hand, one has the ability to influence that prognosis greatly by learning to live with hope and continuing on, without waiting every day to die.

My thoughts returned to my oncologist's voice. He recommended that both chemotherapy and radiation be part of my treatment. The only slight inference to stats was when he said, "Certainly, when we check back with the groups of people who have gone through the treatment program, there are more in that group, and for a longer period of time, than when we check back with the groups of people who have not gone through treatment."

I smiled to myself. I understood the absence of statistical prediction and appreciated that he knew exactly what he was doing in his communication with me. "I would like to have whatever treatment you can give me," I said. "Well, I have two flavours," he said, "Medium and Strong. I would recommend the strongest for your case, but this has to be your decision." I knew that along with the Strong flavour would come Strong side effects. Nevertheless I agreed without hesitation. "Bring in the ground troops!" I said.

From there, both the doctor and the primary nurse began to explain the schedule. It was confusing. There were chemo cycles; some were A's and some were B's, and then there were to be twenty-five sessions of radiation over a five-week period. The chemo would all be done first, and then we'd move on to radiation. There would be intravenous treatments and pills and, of course, we'd need an antibiotic to help stave off infections, although it was most likely that I *would* get an infection, because my blood counts would be so low. There would of course be blood tests to monitor the counts and sometimes if they dipped too low, I would have to delay on more chemo. Consequently, there was no way to predict when all this or that would be completed. And if I got a fever above 37° Celsius I should go immediately to the hospital, because the next morning I could be dead; and there were little charts that I was to fill out each week and bring them back so they could monitor the side effects; and I might be nauseated and would probably need to stay away from salty, spicy and sour foods, but it was very important that I eat to keep my immune system functioning well; and I might *gain weight* because most breast cancer patients did, and . . . sheeeeeeeeeeesh! There was a lot to remember.

The audio on the conversation was tuning in and out, faint and garbled to clear and concise, as thoughts raced through my head. It was like trying to tune into an overseas channel on a fifty-year-old radio that was past its functioning capacity. One of the peripheral things that I remember was when the doctor said something to the effect that when cancer recurs, as in my case, we don't talk so much about a cure, per se, but rather about extending your life for as long as we possibly can and for many people, that can mean years. And by the way, I would be taking Tamoxifen for five years once all my treatment was concluded. And another thing, chemotherapy would activate menopause immediately and I was "most assuredly to lose all my hair, if not within the first treatment, definitely by the second chemo treatment."

The next point that was posed to us was, "Would you like to stay this afternoon and have your first chemo treatment today?" In spite of the flurry going on inside my mind, I was delighted. "Let's get this show on the road," I thought. If he had asked if I would like to put mud all over my face, I would have jumped at the chance. It felt so good to hear so many plans. Action! I liked that. It sure beat sitting around for any more months with this thing inside me gaining strength and speed.

"What about this weight-gain thing?" I asked. I had been secretly hoping that I would *lose* weight on chemo. The last thing that I wanted was to gain more weight. Our culture's value of "young and thin" had made an indelible impression on my sense of self-esteem.

As odd as it may sound, there were times when I didn't know which I was more upset about, having cancer or being overweight. (The Troll would be delighted.) The doctor assured me that there were no calories in the chemo but that for some reason, in spite of mouth sores and nausea most breast cancer patients managed to put on about twelve pounds or six kilos. "Damn, damn!" I thought.

The doctor left the room; the primary nurse stayed with us. She tied up a few more loose ends and was going to arrange the afternoon's appointment in the chemo unit. I was beginning to have misgivings about going into menopause. I wondered if there might be an optional "flavour" that would not cause hot flashes. I asked if she was quite sure that would happen. I wasn't happy about that and my face said so. My "agenda" had always been that I would start menopause at age fifty-five. I had that circled on my mental calendar for some reason and it had been there since I had learned what a menopause was in health class in high school. And here I was, only forty-eight. It threw me. "Oh, come on now," the nurse said. She nudged me in the ribs and jokingly said, "It would have happened soon anyways." She looked to be about the same age as I, and so I decided to let her get away with that remark. "Well, okay," I thought. I guessed that I could make yet another alteration to my agenda. Oddly enough, I was prepared for the announcement that I might lose my hair. All the helpful Cancer Society pamphlets that I had read had equipped me with some good factual information. They had specified that allopecia (hair loss) would not always occur with all chemotherapy. My understanding is that breast cancer therapy is one that does most often cause hair loss.

So I was to gain twelve pounds, lose all my hair, and develop mouth sores and hot flashes. I began to wonder if all my teeth would fall out too. A sarcastic notion! Of course, that does not happen. But it did sound as though I was going to be a fine mess for some time.

Bruce and I went for lunch. Our minds were absolutely swimming. We began to compare notes as to what we had heard and what was to transpire. It didn't take long for us to figure out that we didn't know whether we were coming or going. We did know, however, that we were to be back at the chemo unit for two p.m. That was one detail we had managed to retain.

The thought of an intravenous needle began to cause me great anxiety. My heart was pounding, and a cold sweat began to form on my brow in spite of the hot day. I felt nauseated. I thought about all the gentle little jabs over the past few months from the blood tests, the anaesthetic, the required scanning dyes, and on and on it went. "I'll just have to grin and bear it," I thought, but I was past the point of bravery on that score. I felt that if I saw one more well-meaning person coming at me with a needle to jab in my hand, I would go cowering into a fetal position in a corner somewhere dark where no one could find me ever again.

The Chemo Unit was very large . . . filled with recliner chairs and intravenous poles. We were greeted by warm reassuring staff, who found me my very own recliner and began to set things up. The chemo nurse in charge of my initiation prepared to begin the teaching process for both my husband and me. He sat right there with me through the whole process. It felt good to have my buddy alongside. The first step was to get that IV plugged into me and then we would have a lot to discuss.

The nurse warmed my hand with some hot pads to prepare the veins. What veins? I was half grumbling, half screaming inside myself. Sure enough, no veins would present themselves. No doubt they had taken off for the dark corner where I had planned to escape. Mutiny on the Bounty! Several kind nurses gathered round to inspect the situation. They tried a number of things, but were very perceptive of my fading consciousness and nauseating tension. They disappeared for a consultation. Bruce sat in a chair by my side. I could feel his empathy and his tension. I think he was wishing they would stick the IV into him and then we could get on with things. When the nurses returned a few minutes later, they gently announced that they had talked with my oncologist and that a solution had been found. I was to go to another hospital in a few days to have a PIC line inserted in my arm. It was a semi-permanent catheter to which they would be able to attach the intravenous line. It would remain for the duration of the treatment, and my blood tests could be taken from the same site and all would be well, for me and for them. But for today, they would try to find a vein in my hand, to follow through on the first treatment. I was overjoyed. Suddenly I mustered my reserve courage and let them do the deed.

I wouldn't want to worry future chemo patients about that IV thing. Many folks don't have a PIC line and they make out just great with their good old grass roots veins. My problem was in finding the veins in the first place. The repetitious trial and error to find my veins was the real issue for me.

With that huge barrier out of the way, anything that might come seemed like a piece of cake. The procedure to install the PIC line wasn't that bad. It lasted about ten minutes and was definitely worth investing a little apprehension and anxiety. I was retrofitted with new wheels and ready to journey another thousand miles.

That first teaching session in the chemo unit was expertly done. The chemo pharmacist came out to talk with Bruce and me, and explained all the pills that I was to take and the pills in my kitchen cupboard at home that I was not to take. There were everyday things like the minerals in my vitamins that would interfere with the chemicals of the chemo treatment. There was a lot to learn. Our brains were totally fragmented. But we were given charts and write-ups about everything, so we felt sure we'd be able to figure it all out when we got home. I was overwhelmed by the tension of the day and all the discussions. Bruce stepped in to listen to the instructions and I just sat back and let that wonderful, magical elixir flow through my veins as the IV dripped on. I didn't feel much different. This is going to work just fine, I thought to myself. I was not afraid.

Chapter *8*

Hair Today – Gone Tomorrow

The *priority* on my return home was my head and nothing but my head. Baldness was not likely to be very flattering, I expected. It was a significant concern for me. I went shopping for hats and scarves and was determined that I was going to look good through all this mess if it killed me (well not literally, I hoped). Attractive scarves would be just the ticket, according to the beautiful models that I was seeing in magazines. They looked so exotic. That was my aim. Broad-brimmed hats would come in handy with summer coming up. I had strict instructions that I had to stay out of the sun, considering the sensitivity caused by the medications I would be taking. Long sleeves and garden gloves and big hats were to be the order of the day.

My family stood by patiently as I struggled with accomplishing that "exotic look." I would stand in front of the mirror for hours, tying and retying scarves but never getting it quite right. I seemed to have a little pinhead. This was a new realization and one that I could have lived without. I learned through the "Look Good, Feel Better Program" (offered by the Canadian Cancer Society) that one could use a shoulder pad under the scarf for a fuller-looking skull. Boy, oh boy, I thought. There's a booming new market for shoulder pad manufacturers out there, first in the creation of temporary boobs and now skulls. The tip is a good one. It works for most people.

Finally, I thought I might have accomplished "a look" for myself that wasn't too bad. I ventured downstairs to see what my audience would say. One son greeted me on the fly halfway up the staircase and said, "Oh hi, Mom! That's cute. You look like Aunt Jemima." That was not the review I was looking for. I ventured onward to the kitchen. Bruce turned from the counter, where he was slicing himself some cheese and said, "Well, my goodness, you look like a very attractive cancer patient." I burst out laughing. So did he. "Well, to hell with the scarves," I thought. No matter what I do, I just manage to look like a cross between a pirate or some Yuppie about to do spring cleaning. I just wasn't a scarf girl. But what to do? I couldn't go around bald! I had seen a number of people come into the cancer unit, not the least bit concerned about their bald heads, but I knew that I wasn't that confident or that brave. I still had a full head of hair, but predictions were that this wasn't to last. I was really uptight about looking after this end of my "problem." Bruce looked up Wiggeries in the yellow pages. We didn't have many options in our small city, but there were a few to try out.

The next morning he took me to the mall, and I casually stepped into one of the stores that sold wigs. I had tried one on in earlier weeks at my hairdresser's and looked like Little LuLu, so I wasn't anticipating any great success. But there was one synthetic wig that looked similar to my own hair colour and style. The advice I had received recommended a synthetic wig because they were easy to care for and priced very well.

Wigs are an acceptable claim on many medical insurance plans when accompanied by a doctor's prescription. It seemed like a good deal to me. The sales rep recommended that I first put on a stocking cap (for hygienic reasons in a retail store) and then helped me to get this creature on my head just right. It didn't look too bad. My hopes rose a little. Actually, they rose a lot! "Okay, I'll take it," I said. She looked very pleased about her sale as she watched me remove the wig and then take off the hygienic cap. As I pulled off the tight fitting stocking cap, much of my own natural hair went flying through the air as though someone had blown on a dandelion in full fluff. The whole thing seemed to happen in slow motion. The sales rep and I both looked up in shock and watched as all kinds of hair came floating down through the air. It was only two weeks since I had started my chemo medication. The doctor's words came back to me: "You will *most assuredly* lose your hair, if not in the first cycle, definitely within the second cycle." Boy, the guy in the little giraffe bow tie wasn't fooling around when he made that prediction!

I wasn't upset. I had a great wig to wear. But most of all, I knew that if my hair was falling out, the rapidly dividing cells were dying and that meant that my cancer cells were dying and that was a wonderful, wonderful feeling! It was a jump-start! Such progress and so fast!

I proudly modeled my wig when I returned home. Everyone in the family approved. My other son this time commented, "Boy, that looks even better than your real hair!" and then looked as though he would like to swallow himself when he realized the implications of that compliment. I took no offence. If my wig looked *that* acceptable, I was in business.

Losing one's hair is a messy business, I discovered. I would awaken in the morning with loose hair in my eyes, in my ears and up my nose. A cotton-knit turban proved to be the answer when worn as a nightcap, until all my hair was gone. I read a newspaper article by a famous Canadian author who had breast cancer. She had considered vacuuming her head twice a day during this phase, just to keep things tidy. I was quite amused by the thought of doing such a thing; on the other hand, the idea had merit.

The issue of my balding head was now looked after. Like the PIC line catheter, it was just one more support that was making all this workable and livable for me. It was another stepping-stone along my pathway.

Over the next six months, Bruce and I went to the Chemo Unit twice a month for IV treatments. The sessions took about two hours each and were followed by seven days of chemo pills. Then I would take two weeks off the chemo medication to allow my immune system to build back up before the next session. The program worked in twenty-eight-day cycles. I found there was absolutely no pain involved with this procedure. This was quite contrary to what I had imagined. The chemical program that I would be on was as follows, for the A & B session of each cycle:

Intravenous chemotherapy:
1. Epirubicin, 128 mg.
2. Fluorouracil, 1075 mg (otherwise known as 5FU).

Chemotherapy through pills:

3. Cyclophosphamide, 150 mg per day x 14 days.

Supporting medications during chemo treatment:

4. Dolasetron, 100 mg by IV.

5. Decadron, 8 mg in pill form.

6. Zofran, 8 mg x 3 over a 24-hour period to prevent nausea (pure magic!).

Peripheral medications for my overall health:

7. Ciprofloxacin, 500 mg—an antibiotic to support my immune system's fight in controlling infection.

8. Stemetil—an anti-emetic to prevent nausea as needed throughout the program. I never needed this one.

9. Slow K x 2 per day—introduced later on for a low potassium level.

10. Coumadin, 1 mg daily—a blood thinner needed to keep my catheter line from clogging.

(All vitamin pills and natural remedy pills were retired at the request of the chemo pharmacist to prevent chemical interference with the performance of the chemotherapy.)

I was fascinated to meet other breast cancer patients throughout this time, who were given entirely different mixes of drugs and scheduling. Some days in the chemo unit seemed like "old home week." It was always an interesting character study. We would run into the same people each time and compare notes on types of cancer, individual treatment programs, and progress being made (when known).

On one occasion, we talked with a couple who had been in for treatment often on the same day as my own appointment. She was the patient and he the supporter and translator. Her chemo was causing her to slur her words for some reason. She was an attractive, tiny woman, most likely in her early fifties. I noticed that she arrived in the unit with a little teddy bear under her arm. I found that unusual until she explained that her daughter had bought it for her and named it her Chemo Bear. We talked at length and by the end of the discussion, we learned that she had cancer in her bones, a lung and her liver. After only two months of chemo, her tumours had receded by 50%. She had a very positive outlook. I found this to be exceptional news. I had no idea what activity the cancer was conducting within my lymph nodes but to know that this person was having such great success meant that it was possible for me as well. I was elated all day after hearing that and often found myself thinking about her and wondering what her progress was at different points.

Another couple struck up a conversation with us one day in the waiting room. The woman, her husband, and daughter were from a neighbouring city where I had grown up, so I felt a common link. They looked to be in their sixties, and their daughter would have been about thirty years old. The banter was generally about the upcoming political election, with a few guarded comments about what the future would bring to local constituents if particular parties were to be successful. Since we didn't know their political leanings, we were careful to keep the discussion on a more or less superficial level. Then the woman asked me if this was my first visit. She seemed to be a little shy. I told her that we had been over to the cancer centre several times to date. This was the first for her. "What kind of cancer do you have?" I asked. It seemed ironic to be so comfortable in asking such a personal question of a stranger, when I had not been comfortable at all with the previous political discussion. But because we were there, in this special place where cancer is treated, the formalities around such questions seemed out of place. It was cervical cancer that she had and her doctor felt that they had been very successful in removing it through surgery. But just to be sure, she had been sent over for a single chemo treatment. I compared that to the twelve sessions that I was to have and decided my case must decidedly need chemotherapy. I'm not sure why this was news to me at this point, but there always seemed to be a curiosity inside me about just how serious my situation was. And of course I had not asked my doctor flat out. This kind and quiet woman leaned closer, and whispered to me in a very tentative way, "Do you think we will lose our hair?" I was surprised at the question. I searched the expression on her face, her husband's face and that of her daughter's. It was a serious question. I could tell. "Well, I already have," I said. They sat bolt upright in surprise and then leaned forward again. "Is that a wig?" she asked with an incredulous expression on her face. "Yes, it is," I replied and was feeling just delighted that my wig looked good enough that they had not suspected. I had just assumed that I was sitting there looking spiffy in my new "hair" but that surely the folks in this setting could not be fooled. "Really?" she asked. I assured her that it really was a wig. She was delighted. She looked my hair over very closely and asked me where I had purchased it, and I could see her spirits brighten as she appeared to decide that if wigs looked that good nowadays, she could stop fretting over the possibility of losing her hair.

I felt so good about that all day! I felt good that my wig looked all right, but I felt even better that I had taken the edge off her worries. I could really identify with her concerns. All things being considered, I knew that I would be wearing that thing for about nine months before I had enough hair again to go without it. So getting a good wig had been a very significant support to me.

Some of the time, the Chemo Unit felt akin to being at the hairdresser's, only instead of everyone sitting under hair dryers, we were hooked up to IV poles, and chatting away from our pink-and-blue vinyl-covered recliner chairs. Bruce said it always made him think of sitting down in a restaurant, because the nurse would immediately roll over a tray of goods to be served up. No escargots in garlic butter, though. It was always a tray of sterile gauze, IV bags, carefully labelled medications in big syringes, and tiny sterile pill containers. One day an older gentleman came in and sat down in the big recliner chair beside me. The volunteer, who was also an older good-natured soul, seemed to recognize this patient. She laid out the napkin-like cloth over the arm of his chair, carefully covering his trousers and put some warm packs on his hand to help plump up his veins for the chemo nurse. She lifted his footrest and got a pillow to put behind his head. She was humming away cheerfully. When he was comfy, she clasped her hands together, stood back appraising the situation and said with a twinkle in her eye, "Now sir, can I get you a rum and coke?" I cracked right up! I couldn't stop giggling and neither could he. When we settled down, a few sober moments would pass, and then a snicker would escape from one of us, and we would be into fits of giggles again.

I will always remember the day when a very tall elderly gentleman arrived in the unit with his very tall attractive "thirty-something" daughter holding his arm. They must have each been a minimum of six feet, four inches tall. They were both crying as they walked in. I knew instinctively they had not come for treatments. The nursing team seemed to know them well. I noticed one nurse behind the glass of the nursing station close her eyes in dread and turn her face to the ceiling as if to say, "Oh no, not now, not here." I figured it out without being able to hear the conversation. His wife had been treated for cancer in that very unit, possibly in the same chair that I was sitting in. And she had just passed away that morning. No, no, no, I thought. We, who are sitting here hooked up to these intravenous poles, don't want to see this. We don't want to know about it. Don't you see that I have been meditating and visualizing, and this is not a perspective that fits with my personal plan. But I shed a discreet tear. I could see their anguish. I wasn't angry with them. It brought me momentarily back to a reality check.

At the end of each chemo session, there were hearty interim goodbyes from the folks who were leaving and those still hooked up to their intravenous poles. We were sharing an awesome experience together. There were always silent wishes of good luck. Good luck for you, might mean good luck for me. We're in this together. Stay positive. Stay well. The silent words were spoken by our eyes and our smiles to each other.

Some days, I would see a sad soul come in for treatment and could tell this person was having trouble. The chemo pharmacist would always drop by to visit each of us individually, checking on our medications and how we were feeling. If things were really rough, they were prepared with suggestions and possible adjustments to the chemo treatment as needed. Some folks were quite sick and pale looking. As I listened to them talking with the pharmacist, I could tell they were having a hard time eating and were nauseated most of the time.

I wasn't experiencing this sickness at all and was interested in the fact that other people seemed to be having a difficult time. The one phrase that we heard over and over again, from the doctors and nurses was, *"Every person reacts differently."* They did say that some people just breeze right through chemo and I guessed that I was one of them, in spite of my heavy-duty treatment program. But I couldn't help but feel convinced that the mental preparation I had done, and was still doing, was making all the difference in the world for me.

I was meditating; I was resting; I was freeing myself up from the stresses of everyday life with the tremendous support of my spouse; I was listening to classical music; I was visualizing the chemo as my wonderful, magical ally. Every afternoon I would lie down for a rest and would listen to audio discs to learn how to use the mind/body influence to enhance my immune system. Often I would fall asleep partway through, but my subconscious was still attentively listening, bringing the influence to every cell in my body. The more I listened, the more firmly entrenched the influence became.

I don't mean to say that I felt my usual normal self. There were definitely side effects to my treatment. I began to keep a journal of these side effects. The pattern interested me. In my sharing this, one must remember, *"Every person really does react differently."*

Here are some of the recordings from my own journal and my personal experience:

Chemo Start Date April 28th.   Session 1A

- Felt fine after the first IV—ate supper, no problem; no pureed food for me!

- The muscles in my calves were very sore when I tried to go for a walk the next day, but slowing right down helped.

- The day after IV, my face turned scarlet around noon and it lasted until the next day. This is to be expected. ("Glow-in-the-dark," the nurses called it.)

- No nausea; not very hungry, though.

- Some interesting bowel functions after breakfast and lunch—definitely not a time to delay a visit to the powder room.

- After taking my chemo pills (Cyclophosphamide) on day two and day three of my cycle, my hands and feet went ice cold, but no chills. The doctor had said to watch for chills. This went away after an afternoon nap under our down comforter.

- The morning after IV, I got a hot, itchy feeling that flared up instantaneously on my left ear. The skin seemed dry and peeling. Glycerin and silicone cream took the feeling away instantly. (See Resources.)

- I find that I am walking and generally moving more slowly, but overall I feel okay.
- Not much hunger all week but I am ensuring I eat all my meals to keep my immune system happy. No nausea at all.
- Eating causes hiccoughs if I don't chew very slowly and thoroughly. Orange juice and pineapple juice make me feel sick. Bananas seemed to get stuck partway down after swallowing. Otherwise, all foods are the same as usual. I am not experiencing the taste changes that I have read about.
- Sensitive, red, dry patches developed under my eyes around day six and went away a few days later. The corners of my mouth crack and bleed one day in each cycle but this is easily fixed with a bit of Polysporin.

May   Session 1B

- During the IV session, I started to get a sensation of heartburn in my chest, but it was mild; I also had a dizzy, heavy feeling in my head. (Later on we got to the bottom of this problem and it was eliminated.)
- This is the first IV with the new PIC line catheter. Perhaps it is rushing into my blood stream faster than the natural vein route. The catheter line reaches all the way into a central vein in my chest—I wonder if this is what drug addicts call "mainlining"?
- The nurse slows down the injection of chemo and flushes the line with some solution, and that seems to fix the discomfort.
- Supper is no problem. About 8:30 p.m. a very bad headache surfaces. Not a normal headache. Feels toxic—like a headache I had once when painting with oil-based paint in a small, unventilated room. Not happy about this! Had to lie down and stay very still. Cold cloths on my forehead helped. The toxic feeling went away in about an hour.
- Next day, no issues. No cold hands. HUNGRY—more so than last week.
- I got a headache the second evening but seems like a normal headache; lining of my nose seems to be expanding and taking on a life of its own. Not painful, just unusual.

- Otherwise I feel good.

- May 13th, my hair starts to fall out (day fifteen of chemo).

- Strong allergic reaction to Tegaderm dressings and Transpore tape used for my catheter dressing. Skin blisters badly. Hypofix or Duoderm works well for an alternate. VON nurses are coming in every day to flush the PIC line with a saline solution and look after my dressing. This keeps the line from clogging. They are taking very good care of me.

- During my two weeks off in this first cycle, I find that I am more tired now; low energy during the third week. My blood tests show that my immune system hits rock bottom at the end of the first two weeks and then begins to build again.

- During week four, I feel quite hungry; my energy level is good. I almost feel that I am not on a chemo program.

- Not getting to sleep very easily—low energy but not very sleepy.

June   Session 2A

- There were no uncomfortable sensations when having IV treatment this time.

- On days two and three, my face turned red again; no discomfort with this.

- Very constipated for two or three days but this passes. Prune juice, yuck!

- I feel a real surge in my appetite—hungry all the time—I could eat the furniture! For some reason, I crave ham and cheese sandwiches on bran bread with lots of mayo. And one sandwich is never enough!

- Energy level not too bad—no nausea.

- Gums start to bleed when brushing teeth on days five, six, and seven of the cycle. Rinsing over two days with baking soda and warm water helps clear this up. I bought a "gentle" toothbrush and retired my electric model. Really no mouth sores that were predicted. I think I must be preventing this with my Tea Tree toothpaste. (See Resources.)

- Skin on my face is getting very dry which is unusual for my oily skin. Sore spots under my eyes, but glycerin and silicone cream three times a day helps to resolve this. (See Resources.)

June   Session 2B

- My appetite settles a bit but I am still eating too much!
- Constipation is a big problem on days nine and ten; eating bran and drinking prune juice.
- Shortness of breath on day ten only.
- Quite tired and lethargic. Can't move around quickly.
- Absolutely no nausea. Lost four lbs. at weigh-in ☺
- Days thirteen, fourteen, and fifteen: my gums are bleeding when I brush my teeth.
- I notice that I am getting fine shooting pains occasionally (about twice a month) in my chest where my surgery was. These are the same pains as when my breast was there—like very fine quick currents of lightning—I felt it once this week in my remaining breast. Scary. My body announces that this means something.
- During my two weeks off this cycle, my eyes are sore—not sure if it's the chemo or hay fever. They seem dry. Artificial tears from the drug store are helpful. I wonder if this is a symptom of menopause or a side effect of chemo?
- I have returned to work for mornings only during my two weeks off chemo, with my doctor's consent. It's working out fine as long as I don't move around too much. (The guys on night shift almost fainted when I walked through the door one Sunday evening, with my wig on. I could see they had assumed I was dead, or would be shortly. Hah! Proved them wrong!) The office now seems to be the size of a football field. The hallways that I used to zip up and down, conducting my business many times a day, now seem completely out of reach. I go directly to my office and just stay there. It's a positive boost mentally to be back at work part time and see everybody. It's been three months since I left. I thought I might

never be back. . . . The lineup at my door is heartwarming on the one hand, because people are concerned and want to know if I am all right; on the other hand, they have been badly in need of someone to talk over troubles with in my absence, and it shows.

- Feeling down on day twenty-seven because of fatigue. Gained four lbs.—eating too much ice cream. I sleep a lot in the afternoon.

- No interest in walking. It's too hot out and my wig is like a wool toque. I'm too tired to go walking but worried about gaining weight. Weather is averaging 90°. During week four of this cycle, I notice the cheeks of my face getting larger. They said that would happen from the steroid that I take on IV day. . . . Moon face! Just what I need! Is it just my imagination?

This week and last week, my feet are not working well—very stiff for two or three minutes when I get up to walk. Find myself hobbling until they become flexible again. Legs very stiff and achy if I stand for a while cooking.

July   Session 3A

- The night of day one, I eat supper with no problem. My head feels slightly "nauseated." After supper, the "nauseated head" increases but not a huge problem—no desire to snack (good thing). My head feels thick—slightly off balance—no quick head movements, please!

- My feet continue to be very stiff and are starting to feel all bruised inside, but I notice this does not happen during the two weeks *on* chemo—only the two weeks that I am *off* chemo. That's puzzling. The doctor doesn't know what is causing this.

- Eating too much! Is it the steroids that are making me hungry?

July   Session 3B

- Nauseated head again the day of IV treatment—like a huge hangover.

- No problems with my feet this week
- I have experienced dizziness for an hour or so during two days of both sessions 3A and 3B.
- Feel that my brain is quite "wired" after IV—lots of busy creative thoughts—could this be the steroids? I lay awake all night thinking of interesting and colourful things. Not depressed.
- My eyesight seems to be deteriorating; the sunlight bothers my eyes; words are very blurred when reading and usual glasses are not helpful. Bought some drugstore reading glasses for the end of my nose. Look like a granny—but they work.
- My feet are causing me problems again. Surgical Pathology Report says that my cancer is "highly suspicious for vascular invasion"—is this what is wrong with my feet? Is this what caused me so much fatigue last year? The doctor says that cancer doesn't show up as fatigue. This puzzles me.
- Find that I am feeling more and more tired. The chemo seems to be having a cumulative effect on my energy level.
- Have lost 90% of my eyebrows and eyelashes these last two weeks. How insulting! My blue eyes remind me of a Siamese cat, naked of lashes and brows. Strange look—makes me very self-conscious. Have to learn to draw on eyebrows, just like Roger Rabbit's girlfriend. Geeeee whiz!
- Skin on my face is not as dry. Able to settle my appetite with concerted effort.
- Lots more energy from day twenty-five to twenty-eight of this cycle—not back to normal, but better.
- My face seems puffy—feet, too.
- *I figure out that my Cipro (the antibiotic prescribed to help me fight infection when my immune system is deteriorating) is the culprit when mixed with my chemo on intravenous day. Eliminating the Cipro on that day only eliminates the toxic headache! Hallelujah!*
- Those previously advertised hot flashes are here. Seem to occur mainly in the morning when I am trying to get ready for work.

Applying makeup to a sweaty face is frustrating and this seems to intensify the hot flash. But I need my makeup. Otherwise I look like a cancer patient!

There were six cycles of two IV treatments each, in total, over a period of five months. As time wore on, I could feel the effect of the chemo accumulating in some respects. My fatigue continued and the annoying abuse of my feet continued off and on. In other respects, my body was adjusting to the drugs and many of the side effects just went away. I was really coping quite well.

Finally we noted that I had only two more chemo sessions to go. The countdown began. The mere mental boost of being "almost through" began to pay good dividends to my overall feeling. I was looking forward to growing hair again, getting my catheter out and perhaps feeling well enough to go walking in the nice fall air. I thought I should be planning to jump out of a cake, in celebration! I knew that I had yet to do twenty-five sessions of radiation over a five-week period, but nonetheless, a milestone had been reached. I didn't feel as though I were inside a tunnel anymore.

On the Monday of my last chemo week, I began to worry about the final visit with my VON nurse. A team of nurses had been covering my case for the five-month period, first coming in every day and then later dropping that back to three visits a week. They did a superb job of ensuring that my health was not any further complicated throughout this vulnerable period. There was one nurse in particular that Bruce and I had instinctively bonded with. She seemed to be the lead for my case and was the one we most frequently saw. Her competence, her unfaltering, conscientious approach was consistent, even on a hot summer day with a demanding schedule of patients to be met. She was always very particular to ensure that things were going just right with my catheter and with my overall wellbeing.

She involved my husband in my care. He was the "blood runner." Every day prior to IV treatments, blood samples would have to be drawn and rushed to the hospital's lab to ensure my blood counts could be determined in time for the formal go-ahead for the chemo treatment the following day. If they had dropped too low, chemo would be postponed. We named him Count Dracula and our dog Woody was a major shareholder in that transportation function as well. Gwen (my nurse) had allowed Woody to bond with her and that endeared her even more closely to us.

Gwen arrived again on the Wednesday of that week for "Bloody Wednesday." This was to be her last visit. As she was finishing up all the required functions of her role, we were chatting and packing up the medical supplies. I felt my eyes welling up with tears and was trying to hold back. I had read about patients getting attached to their medical teams through such a life-threatening experience. On an intellectual level, I didn't want to be grouped in with those folks, simply because I understood what was happening. Silly pride. On the other hand, I felt such gratitude to this nurse for the immaculate care that she and the others on the team had given to me. And besides, we both liked her very much as a person. In other circumstances, she would have become a good friend, and that's not a decision I make lightly. I choose to have few friends, but the ones I have are very close to me.

I cried. I made her cry. "I hope that if I see you again," I said emphatically, "it will be in the grocery store." Then I added on a more serious note, that if I ever became sick again, I hoped she would be my nurse. We blew our noses with large paper towels, had a giggle and a hug and parted company.

I sat there quietly in our living room and wondered to myself if it would really be over, or if this was only the beginning.

Chemotherapy had begun on April 28th, some five months earlier. September 24th was to be my last treatment at the hospital Chemo Unit and would be followed by seven days of chemo pills at home. The nurse administered my chemo as efficiently as always. He was a warm, friendly fellow with a jovial sense of humour. After a few hours, my husband went out for a stretch and to take Woody out of the car for a whiz. Woody always came with us—the Three Musketeers. As I was chatting with the nurse, I got up the nerve to ask him about one of the other patients; a subject that I was concerned might be taboo. I didn't want to be a nosey neighbour and was conscious that he would be bound by ethical confidentiality. I asked tentatively, "I noticed that I haven't seen Mr. So-and-So and his wife in here the last while. Is she still coming for chemo?" This was the lady with the little chemo bear, the one whose tumours had receded by 50% after only two months. The nurse hesitated and then said quietly, "She passed away two weeks ago." "Oh," I said, and he finished up the last of his chemo procedures. Both of us were silent. For some reason, I had known the answer before I asked the question. I didn't want to talk anymore. When Bruce returned, I told him about it. "Oh, gee," he said, and looked very sad. He didn't want to talk about it, either.

This was also the day I would have my PIC line catheter removed. I had had tubes coming out of me for various reasons for over six months now. I was so excited about losing that darn thing, even though it had served me well and been a great support to all those IV treatments. Removing that last stitch holding the catheter squeaked a split-second yelp out of me, but the removal of the line caused no pain at all, even though it was over a foot long. My body was now my own again, minus a part, but still mine.

I made rice pudding that night in celebration of the milestone. Bruce had been asking me for my famous rice pudding for two years and I was always too busy or too tired to make it for him. We ate one batch and then I made another one. I was still on chemo pills so we couldn't exactly break open a bottle of wine. We also conducted a humorous ceremony, complete with verbal drum roll and disposed of the remainder of my Coumadin pills, the blood thinner required by the dearly departed catheter. "Won't need those puppies anymore," I thought to myself in delight. I then eyed the kitchen cupboard stocked with the remainder of my chemo pills and peripheral pill bottles needed as support through the chemo and thought how nice it would be next week, when I could trash them all.

I was finding myself frequently wondering if this would be the end of it. I wondered how safe I would be without that magic elixir running through my system.

My last day on chemo was a day of bitter and sweet.

Chapter 9

Insight Lost, Insight Gained

So much more evolved through that five-month period of chemotherapy. If the truth were known, I think it was I who evolved. I found my inner spirit—the centre of my soul. It was a place that I had never really been to before in my entire lifetime.

I had always thought of myself as a pawn placed on the game board of life. I felt separate from life itself in many ways, an observer of myself, as I moved through the stages of my life. I felt a deep connection with the other pawns, bishops, kings and queens on the game board, the people of my life. But I felt little or no connection between myself and nature, the world, and the universe.

As I looked into the kaleidoscope of my life, the colours fragmented into millions of sizes and shades and shapes. The pattern was continuously changing before my eyes: my life and motherhood, my life and my kindred spirit, my life and my education, my life and career, my life and my parents, my life and friends, my life and my business relationships, my life and my past, my life and my future, but rarely my life and my present moment.

It was all badly out of balance, I suspected. Each of the dimensions of my world was composed of contradictory tensions. Even when I was at rest physically, my mind raced onward, in and out of the ever-widening networks and demands that expanded like the spinning of a vastly complicated spider web.

And in spite of the fact that I had cancer, life moved onward. One son graduated from high school and left a few short months later to attend university. This was a momentous turning point in my life, to give him up to the world. But we left him on the threshold of a very big adventure, and the pure excitement of that, as well as the twinkle of anticipation in his eyes, helped to soothe the pain of separation I was feeling. Thank goodness I still had one twin at home for the next year. I could let them go in stages and hoped that the world would not be ripped from under my feet when the remaining dear soul made his way into the next phase of his life as well. It seemed like yesterday that the boys were running through the house, chasing the dog with their little jammy hands, sometimes laughing, sometimes screaming, sometimes crying. Whatever the dilemma, I always felt that I was experiencing motherhood in stereo with one twin in my right ear and the other in my left. It was non-stop and I would think that when the day came for university, I would lovingly say with a great sigh of relief, "It's been a wonderful experience. Love ya! See ya!" I never suspected that the attachment and my need to be a necessary part of their lives as their mother would grow so completely and profoundly that it would be this hard to let go.

In the outer world, mass shootings were unleashed by disturbed people in both Canada and America; and to top it all off, John F. Kennedy Jr., his wife and her sister died in that fateful plane crash that broke hearts all over the world. We often held our breath when turning on CNN and saw the frequent "Breaking News!" alert on the screen. On the home front, my mother and I chatted long distance every weekend, Bruce accomplished an active and successful golf season, and my son who remained in the nest was successful in landing his first real part-time job. The tension in our household that week while he prepared for the job interview was unreal. When he finally got the acceptance call we were delighted for him. It was a happy milestone.

Shortly thereafter, the boys' paternal Nanny died. She had been a strong and influential matriarch on that side of the family. I found the funeral especially difficult. Death was something I didn't want to think about and it seemed only a short while ago that I had been in the same church over my daughter's death. Ten years had not softened that memory for me. My son Christopher did the eulogy for his grandmother and it was a masterful moment in his life that touched our hearts forever.

All of this occurred within the five months that I was on chemo. I was tempted to go out into my back yard and get up on a box and shout over the fence at God and the world, "Breaking News! I have cancer, you know! How dare life continue on! Could you not have the decency to press the Pause button, at least until I am out of this chasm and can catch up with the rest of you?" But the thought was a fleeting one.

I cancelled it out on the realization that I was very grateful that life was moving onward. "And so must I," I thought to myself.

Looking back over the past year, I considered all the unforeseen events that had transpired and wondered: what will the next year bring to our lives? New Year's Eve would bring in the Millennium. That feeling of foreboding crept slowly up the back of my neck again. It seemed to appear and disappear as illusively and unexpectedly as a ghost.

Everything that I was purposefully reading had a connection to wellness and spiritualism. Very unusual topics for me, who usually had my head buried in an organizational development textbook! I marvelled at the peace these insights brought to my mind and knew they were doing me a world of good in more ways than dealing with my cancer. New thoughts, new insights and new behaviours were entering my life, replacing the demands of business and financial concerns for the future and that hurry-up mental schedule of mine. It was soothing a long-standing internal and unconscious heartburn.

I learned how important it was to go outside and stand on the lawn in my bare feet, to feel the earth beneath me, to wiggle my toes in the grass and feel the sun on my face and to understand that my body and my soul were the extension of a much larger universe of which I was very much a living, breathing part. I began to feel that I was an important part of the universal system and not just an observer, a pawn on a chessboard. I made a very concentrated effort to live IN the moment, to appreciate it thoroughly with nothing else on my mind. I would sit alone on the sundeck in the early morning, studying the two maple trees that we had carefully dug up from the ski hill in the spring, when they were just budding as baby trees. They had grown so tall and full in these past five years and to me they represented the vibrant growth that our family shared together. And after a time, the leaves of the trees would slowly come into focus. The sun would shine through and varying shades of green would become rich and warm and alive, as though a 3-D camera were bringing the picture into exceptional focus for my eyes. I could see it so clearly that the warmth of the experience touched deeply inside my mind and my soul. How many times had I sat in that same chair before, looking outward, looking at the same maple trees, looking past them but never really seeing them? And now the rustle of the leaves would fill my ears and I felt a comfort from them as though they were a part of my body and I of theirs. I smiled to myself thinking of an insightful thing that Linus had once dryly said: "Don't be a leaf, Charlie Brown, BE A TREE!" How profound!

It was like arms surrounding me to keep me safe from harm in life or perhaps, I realized, in death. The experience was deeply sensory and etched itself into my soul.

A most cherished time during these five months, was the day my spouse decided he would renew my spring garden for me. My garden is a very treasured experience and one that I came upon only about five years ago. Gardening had never really been of interest to me until we moved to this home and began to make the small plot of land our own. It was an interest that Bruce and I shared. He taught me to cultivate the soil, to fertilize it, to plant my new treasures with enough space for growth and to prepare it for winter's sleep. My flower garden is like a community of personalities that I plant and watch grow, always delighted with the changes and surprises that unfold. My flowers have personalities just like people; some are shy, some aggressive, some are precocious and some are good old stable standbys. Some flowers have trouble and need extra nurturing to help them be the best they can be. They seemed like children that needed to be nurtured and responded beautifully to care and love and kindness. I had spent many hours poring over garden books, planning the colours and textures and timing of the blooms that would become part of my treasure chest.

But this year I was not strong or well enough to do a lot of bending and digging, and I was silently stewing about what would happen to my garden. My pink-and-blue calico print garden gloves were hanging on a nail in the garage, not used since summer past but covered in the soil from last year's planting and definitely shaped to the form of my own hands. My spouse picked up on my concern seemingly by osmosis and announced that he would spiffy up my garden for me. I was elated! In late May, we went to my small plot down by the fence of our backyard and assessed the state of the nation. Even though I couldn't participate to any great extent, I wanted to be there with him.

I sat on the grass and waited for the clumps of undergrowth that he would pile up as he pulled and dug the dead growth away to make room for the new spring life that was timidly beginning to surface. He would dig and I would put the spent leaves and plants into a garbage bag for removal. Those bad raspberry plants were creeping under the fence from our neighbour's crop again this year, pesky things, full of fine nettle that I dared not get in my hands in case of infection. My depleted immune system cautioned me on taking such a risk. He yanked them all out, to my delight.

The new plants that we had purchased were waiting in their little pots to join the larger community of my garden. Planting flowers represents new life to me—I felt that a new beginning was being planted especially for me. As Bruce weeded the garden, I identified with the process as though it were purging the cancer from my body. That golden sunny day that my husband cleaned up all the undergrowth and cultivated the soil, expanding and clarifying the edging of my garden, felt like a new lease on life for me. I sat in the shade under our maple trees for the first time, a newfound discovery that had not previously occurred to me. All my medication precluded my sitting in the sun. Woody stretched out his long furry body on the cool grass beside me, rolling around and scratching his back with a silly expression of ecstasy on his little upside-down black face.

I was planning the new lilies that would be just the right thing for the blank spot at the back. That had been bothering me. I didn't like blank spots in my garden. It was an eclectic collection of this and that and the other thing. I liked to think of it as an English garden. Many of the plants represented endearing memories to me, the two rose bushes that our daughter and son-in-law had given me for Mother's Day, the pink prairie mallow that my son had given me for my birthday, the hollyhock from my other son's original first garden that he had created at about age fourteen; and then there was the garden stone of Christopher's large, friendly handprint—a bear paw at age nineteen. I didn't necessarily like a lot of predefined order to the plantings. But something in that blank spot was lost, not quite right. Planning for next summer's show felt good; I would be here to see it and that was part of the plan as well. My mind was taking me forward unconsciously to the days ahead when I would be completely well.

My favourite flower in the garden was the Echinacea, or purple coneflower, as many know it. I thought back to the visualization therapy I had been doing after my surgery, when the snow still lay on the ground, and recalled the segment where I was to think of myself as a flower seed being planted into the rich black earth, within my own body. As I sat and watched the process of my garden's spring renewal, I pictured myself again as an Echinacea plant, starting out as a little seed and slowly reaching my arms and leaves up to the warm sunlight, stretching upward, growing tall and very strong, with firmly planted roots, beautiful velvety purple petals and formidably spiked copper-coloured stamens at the centre of each of my flowers. The Echinacea plant is said to heal the immune system. I believe it. We take Echinacea tincture drops through the winter, whenever we feel a cold coming on and miraculously cure the cold before it even gets out of the starting gate. I said to Bruce as he cultivated the rich soil, "Someday, I would like to come back to this world as an Echinacea plant." He looked at me and then quietly returned to his turning of the soil. The pink-and-orange sherbet parrot tulips were in full bloom and the *Fritillaria* stood like tall inverted yellow jester's caps in the centre of my garden. Every time I looked at them, they laughingly said to me, "Don't worry, be happy!" My Echinacea plant would not be in bloom until late July but it didn't matter, since it grew strong and tall within me as it helped to heal my body. My dear husband cared for me throughout my sickness as he cared for my garden that day.

When Jordan graduated at the end of June, I was well enough to attend the ceremony with the rest of the family. Bruce's daughter, my chosen daughter, would be there as well. I wanted to look nice for my son. It was an important day. All reports were that the gymnasium would be very hot; there was no air conditioning. I was in a stew about that, never having liked the heat and now filled with chemo drugs and sporting a woolly wig, I wasn't sure how I would manage. That sort of environment usually left me wilted and crabby. As I applied my lipstick and blush in the mirror that morning, I stepped back and looked at the foreign face in the mirror. My head was entirely bald, except for five kinky sparse hairs that persisted on hanging in there. Most people would have gotten a buzz cut before losing all their hair, but I couldn't be bothered. I looked like the Grinch from Doctor Seuss; no hair, no eyebrows and no eyelashes. I had purchased a wide-brimmed straw hat during my strategic planning for hair loss. This was to be part of my outfit for the big day. I put on a special dress and beautiful long silk scarf that my mother had sent to me. My brushed silver dangling earrings looked to be of aboriginal descent and had lots of quiet, tasteful personality. The hat would just complete my outfit nicely. I intended to look terribly chic. But to my surprise, when I put it on, the hat dropped below the bottom of my nose and ears! I gasped and then realized that with my hair gone, the fit was an entirely different proposition. I began to giggle and couldn't stop; this seemed the stuff that cartoons are made of. The wig would have to do. In spite of this mishap, the graduation ceremony created significant memories that we were able to share as a family. I was glad to be here to take part in the day, a special moment in my son's life.

Returning to work in July alleviated the boredom that was beginning to set in after three-and-a-half months of relaxation. Things had changed a lot at the office. The first major restructuring had gone full circle after our merger and people had just started to climb out of the trough of stress and depression. It was wonderful to see everyone and for the first few days I had a steady stream of visitors at my office door, checking in to see how I was and checking in to chat and let me know how they were after the recent restructuring. Their tired faces looked weary and troubled. I realized that their journeys and mine were running as parallel challenges.

One of the managers with whom I had worked over the past two years had been "downsized" last January, but came into the office for a short visit with everyone. One positive side of traditionally paternalistic companies is that they create a family bond between people that is hard to break. Unfortunately, along with that comes a dependence on that company to keep people safe from all woes. As a result, the pain is much more significant when historically unprecedented layoffs begin to occur. It's like severing the umbilical cord. The sunnier side of this evolution was that the majority who were close enough to bridge to their pension, were left with a grin from ear to ear. But even for them, it took a few months to adjust to the idea that their thirty-plus-year careers would not extend into the future of the new organization. But my, what a purposeful and colourful legacy they were leaving with us! A legacy that was crafted from their own blood, sweat and tears.

This "downsized" manager hadn't been gone two months before he ended up in hospital with a terrible *E. coli* infection in his eye—one of only ten cases in the world. As I sat looking at him across my desk he told me of his experience. After months in the hospital, the infected eye had been removed in order to rescue the other eye. He had a positive and accepting attitude and was adjusting well. There were many things to think of, however, including adjustments in driving and walking, and so much more. I thought of my breast that had been removed and noted to myself that I would much rather have lost a breast than an eye. I nudged him in the ribs, and suggested that we do a road show throughout our organization, he with his artificial eye and I with my artificial breast and we laughed at the prospect of this.

So much had changed. So many people were gone to early retirement. In some ways, my once familiar surroundings seemed like a ghost town. Phil had lost his eye, I had lost my breast, Joey had died of cancer last month, and two more of our employees were now in the hospital with colon cancer and who knew what would become of them.

I wasn't back at work long before the corporate office announced that another big shakeup would be coming so as to implement further restructuring. That meant more layoffs and the staff knew it. They were battle-worn and easily thrust into despair about what the future would bring. We seemed to be trapped in an unfortunate revolution of organizational history that I felt sure we

would be reading about in textbooks in the years to come. I thought
of a little poem I had read in one of my "change management" books:

> *"There is one fault that I must find*
> *With the twentieth century,*
> *And I'll put it in a couple of words:*
> *Too adventury.*
> *What I'd like would be some nice dull monotony,*
> *If anyone's gotony."*

Ogden Nash

Good God, the organizational changes were having a dramatic
impact on people! I was glad to be there to help out, I was glad of the
intellectual stimulation and the challenges to be met; but at the end
of each two-week period, I was awfully glad to step out of it all and
to go home to my fuzzy slippers and my peaceful cancer treatment
program. I began to worry about how I would continue in the work
world for at least another ten years and not allow myself to get
sucked back into the quicksand of stress that was so inherent in
organizational life at that time. Non-stop mergers and acquisitions
seemed to be happening in most large companies everywhere. It was
an epidemic akin to the surge of cancer throughout the population. I
had to make a pact with myself that I was to come first. I would no
longer drag home that heavy briefcase full of unfinished work. I
would leave the house in the morning with my lipstick in my pocket
and that was the only thing I would drag home with me at night.

Simplifying one's outer style of living is key to a successful
recovery. But it's really the inward simplicity that changes one's life. I
had worn so many pairs of shoes over the years. I stepped in and out
of them as I grew and as the occasion warranted—the shoes of
ambition, the shoes of competition, the shoes of accumulation of
material possessions, the shoes of pride and ego, the shoes of survival.
This footwear was becoming less necessary as my priorities began to
shift and as I moved into a new phase of my life. Finding my true
centre was something I had to do alone; no one else could do it for
me. I was intent on feeding my soul.

One night, early on in my chemo treatment, one of those creative steroid-kind-of-nights, I lay in bed staring at the dark ceiling. It was three a.m. and I had not yet been able to sleep. I found myself thinking about my life and my work—my usual busy brain activity. I don't think that I was asleep, but I might have been dreaming. I could see myself in the boardroom at my company's local office. I was facilitating a meeting with the management team. As I stood at the flip chart, a cold, fierce wind began to steal its way through the room. The papers on the table were whisked away, the pictures on the walls were sucked up into the air, the lights went out and finally one by one, each manager around the table disappeared into thin air. It seemed like a Stephen King movie, the kind I was always too frightened to watch. I found myself whirling through the dark night. When I woke up, I was crouching naked on the floor of a dense forest. The dark fir trees seemed to reach right up to touch the sky. It was very dark, rainy and cold. I shivered in the night air. I wasn't frightened, but I was completely stunned.

"*What is the purpose of your being?*" was the question being asked of me, over and over again. I couldn't tell if the question was coming from the trees, from the air, from some other being, or from within myself. I didn't know the answer. "*If you were to leave this world at this moment, what contributions have you made? Have you done everything you could possibly do with the body and the mind that you were given?*" The questions kept coming in a loud insistent whisper. I didn't know the answer. I hadn't really ever thought about these things.

The answer to the questions came to me very quietly. There was no drum roll, no bash of symbols. I realized that the answer was there all along, the night the questions were being asked. I just had to clear the way so that I could hear it. But it wasn't really a matter of hearing. It was a matter of quietly and surely knowing. I wanted more time and connection with the people that I love—my family. I had been consumed throughout my career of twenty-five years with improving myself as a professional. I wanted now to focus more on the present—to live IN the moment and enjoy it. I wanted to stop pressuring myself to become everything and to try everything. I wanted to find balance in every aspect of my life. I wanted inner peace. And most of all, I wanted to help the people that I care about, in my family and my work, to be happy and at peace within themselves. *This was my purpose for being.* It was good to have the answer—so simple and yet so hidden from me all this time. It was something I had been too busy to hear my whole adult life.

Looking back over the five months of chemo, it had really not been so bad. It was not nearly the nightmare that I had anticipated. It seemed that having faith, for me, meant giving up control. There was no longer a need for Denial. When I would get to the end of my rope, instead of clinging desperately to it, I would reach out and trust that something new would come in its place. It was like swinging from one trapeze to the other, knowing fully well that there was a safety net below. I didn't have to do it all alone. When I found myself struggling with something, I learned to let it go for the moment and trust that there was a greater source holding it for me. This allowed me to rest, to relax my grip, to breathe new life into myself. And the answers would follow. It's very hard to hear your inner spiritual guidance when you are holding on so fiercely that you can't breathe and listen. I had been too busy for years and years to really listen.

My son-in-law asked me one night at dinner after some insightful reading, "Are we all human beings having a spiritual experience or are we really spiritual beings having a human experience?" (Myss, 1996). He is a very bright individual and I was glad to hear that he had uncovered such a question this early in his life. I wondered why it had taken me so long to see the point.

Chapter 10

Untold Secrets Of The Daffodil
Terrace Lodge

October presented itself in shades of burnished gold, russet, cinnamon, orange and red. The air was clear and crisp and most often illuminated by blue skies warmed with vibrant golden sunshine. Colour surrounded Bruce and me like an autumn patchwork quilt covering us warmly before the long winter's snow would anaesthetize the countryside. Huge rock cuts on either side of the highway stood as sentinels that we were to pass through many times in the next five weeks. The transition from summer to fall seemed to announce the arrival of the final phase of my treatment program.

Our two-hour monthly drive to the cancer centre would now become a weekly expedition through the glory of nature's fall season. The radiation I was to receive could not be done in our hometown. And since the program required five treatments each week, Monday to Friday, over five weeks, it now became necessary to leave my family to stay in a neighbouring city at the Daffodil Terrace Lodge, a wing of the cancer treatment centre. There would be many other cancer patients. It sounded depressing. I didn't want to go, but I did dearly want the additional insurance that radiation might provide to ridding my body of cancer.

"Five weeks is not really as long as the five months of chemo I have just been through," I told myself. Even so, it was difficult to tear myself away from home, my cocoon, to stay with strangers and pass the time with activities that really had no appeal in the first place.

Meredith, a sharp young volunteer student, had taken us on a tour of the Daffodil Terrace Lodge some weeks before. I had to admit, it was a beautiful and comfortable facility that really didn't have any remote resemblance to a hospital, even if it was attached to the cancer centre. My room was comparable to anything a well appointed hotel would have to offer, decorated as it was in washed oak furniture, wonderfully huge windows, and soft shades of rose and heather green. There were no bedpans, no privacy curtains or side rails around my bed, no fluorescent lighting. There were two lockable closets with lots of shelving and places to hang clothes, a conclusive indicator that I was to share a room with someone else: a fact that I was not comfortable with. But I supposed that I could go along with the program.

There were five floors to the lodge, each with a comfy TV room to be shared. The third and fourth floor TVs were reserved for sports only. There were laundry facilities for guest use on the third floor and a large dining room on the first floor where guests would gather throughout the day for meals and activities. In the basement, we found a billiards room and a great library with wall-to-wall books, a computer, and a magnificent large-screen television for movies, complete with an extensive collection of videos. Someone had planned this place very carefully, thinking of every detail that one might want if one had to be away from home for an extended period.

I had noticed during the tour that Monday night was for Sing Along, Tuesday night was Bingo night, and Wednesday was Craft Day; and to each one of those special events, I thought, "Not for me," "not for me," and "not for me."

"They'll probably want to make me do basket weaving," I snorted to myself. And I would be damned if I was going to play bingo, of all things! Being a loner at heart, the mere thought of group activities raised my hackles. I love people, but having the option to have my own space when I need some "down time" is very important to me, and there were likely to be a lot of cheery people telling me how good it would be for me. I also don't enjoy a lot of administrative rules, and this place looked so well organized and spotlessly clean that I expected there would be some head person with a long list of annoying rules that I would need to grumble about. Five weeks looked like five years, and a dull feeling in the pit of my stomach began to settle in.

Bruce had decided long before my arrival at the Lodge that he would like to stay with me the first night, if that were possible. He marketed the notion that he needed to see where I would be and know what would go on there so that he could feel comfortable himself. But I suspected all along that he was trying to help me to make the transition smoothly. We were joined at the hip; a separation of this kind would create more than just a blip on the screen. Since a roommate had not yet been assigned, the second bed in my room was available, and the staff were agreeable to having an additional guest for one night. I was very relieved that he would be with me. We explored the Lodge, went out for dinner and played pool in the billiards room that evening and quite enjoyed ourselves. My first day there was a Thursday and, with the onset of the weekend, all guests were planning to travel home for a break. They would return on Monday for another week of daily radiation appointments. I was glad of Bruce's company and very pleased to be going home with him the next day. It helped me to ease into a foreign and not-so-welcome land.

The initial days in radiation were technically fascinating to me. An "alpha cradle" had to be made to provide support to my body for each of the twenty-five sessions. Three technicians helped to create the customized pillow. I lay on a table with a bare chest, putting arms and hands above my head, allowing my form to create its shape in a soft plastic pillow that seemed to be filled with small foam beads. Once comfortable, the air was either removed from the pillow with a hose or some substance was infused into the pillow. I wasn't quite sure what happened, but the end result was like a plaster-of-Paris form that molded right to my head, neck, shoulders and arms.

The technicians also made the preparations for a "dry run" that was to occur the next day. I was hearing a lot of mathematical equations being bandied about as they measured my chest from what seemed like hundreds of angles, drawing X's and dashed lines and dots with magic marker across the left side of my chest, where there had once been a breast. There were measurement rulers in every shape. The technicians' gentle voices were discussing things above my outstretched body, each time explaining the process to me and apologizing for their cold hands. I was completely mesmerized by their work. Once all the angles and measures had been taken, some very tiny permanent tattoo marks about the size of a freckle were dotted on my skin. These were to be locators for the radiation therapists, who would be carefully lining my body up each day to ensure that the radiation would enter my body at the planned strategic angles. When I looked at my chest that evening in the bathroom mirror, I was amused with all the colourful ink drawings. They resembled a blueprint for city hall. I was to leave all markings on, wherever possible, for the full five weeks.

The next day, I was briefed by a radiation therapist regarding the care of my skin during and after radiation. I was not to use soap, deodorant, lotions or anything that would add chemicals to my skin in the area that was to be radiated. Johnson's Baby Powder or cornstarch would keep my skin dry and smooth throughout the treatment. I was told that I might get a very sore throat and that the radiation would include my chest, underarm and collarbone area to ensure the lymph nodes were dealt with. The sore throat never did materialize. The therapist anticipated that I would have a skin reaction similar to sunburn about two weeks into the treatment. Being very fair-skinned, I assumed the burn would be significant for me. I remembered extensive blistering as a child who loved to stay out in the sun and the water far longer than was healthy. The therapist's final prediction was that because radiation causes fatigue and since I had already been through five months of chemo, I might expect to feel like a wet noodle partway through the program. None of the anticipated side effects concerned me all that much after my adventures with chemo. We were ready for the dry run and then it was home for the weekend.

That first Friday morning, I noticed the lobby of the lodge was all a-twitter with activity. People were scurrying around with looks of delightful anticipation on their faces. Suitcases were packed and waiting beside each owner—waiting for a driver from the Cancer Society to come and chauffeur their respective groups home for the weekend to be with their families. Some would travel in vans to communities as far as six hours away. Every Friday morning would carry this excitement at the Lodge. It was like being part of a wired-up group of kids on Christmas morning.

The following Monday, we traveled our now familiar route along the highway and back to the cancer centre. I didn't notice the colourful scenery on this trip, except to take in the fact that it was cold and the sun wasn't shining, no doubt to add credence to my gray mood. My thoughts were elsewhere. My bags were packed with enough clothes and books, and I had my laptop computer. I had packed carefully with five weeks of boredom and loneliness in mind. I knew that I would be going home again every weekend, but five weeks was still five weeks, 5 weeks, *five weeks,* V weeks. I would much rather have been on my own sofa, under my blanket and inside my introverted turtle shell. I could chat with my son and my husband, the dog would be at my side, and Oprah would be hosting my favourite program on television.

But instead, Bruce and I would arrive at the Daffodil Terrace Lodge, unpack my belongings, have lunch together and shortly thereafter, say goodbye to each other. I watched him drive off and felt an overwhelming wave of loneliness wash over me. I lay on my bed most of that afternoon, looking out the window at the gray fall skies and wished that I could somehow fast-forward to the end of the week, when he would come to get me again. It was a very long and silent afternoon. There would be no roommate for a few days, which suited me just fine. I could be as gloomy-glum as I damned well pleased.

By five p.m. my hunger got the best of me. I would have to venture out, navigate my way through the Lodge and into the unfamiliar hallways of the cancer centre to the adjoining hospital cafeteria. The food selections looked pretty decent and there were several tables at which I could choose to sit alone. I didn't feel like making conversation today. Another time, perhaps. I made my way back to my room and read for most of the evening, falling into an early but restless sleep. The bed was not my bed, there was no one to snuggle up to and I hated the pillow. The next morning when I woke up, I was still there at the damned Daffodil Terrace Lodge with five weeks still stretching ahead of me. The night's sleep had not altered my situation in any way.

Coffee was the consuming priority on my mind. I floated to the lobby in the elevator about seven a.m. and was greeted by the cheery staff on the front desk. They needed to see me in the office, to take my blood pressure and capture the list of medications I was taking. I was gently surprised by the reminder that the "front desk" types at this hotel were really nurses dressed in professional business attire rather than in medical uniforms. They were fully qualified and equipped to handle any potential "guest" needs. During my stay, I would become familiar with their individual and beautiful dispositions, their professionalism and their warm humour. They skilfully set the tone and spirit for the overall Lodge, like a finely balanced thermostat subtly regulating the comfort level of a home during adverse weather.

I made my way to the dining room of the Lodge for breakfast. Guests were invited to bring their own groceries and to prepare their meals in the kitchen area of the dining room. I had decided this would be a good option, at least for breakfast. Cafeteria scrambled eggs were not something to live and breathe for, I presumed. There were microwave ovens, toasters, dishes, and an extensive refrigerator that accommodated the individually labelled boxes of goodies each resident had brought for their stay. There was a lot of buzz going on in the dining room. People were clustered at different tables, making plans for the day. Other than our thirty-minute appointments with radiation occurring at different intervals each day, our time was to be our own.

A tall, gray-haired lady, with a presence of intelligence and authority, stepped right up to me and said, "You must be new." She was reading my nametag without my permission, I thought as I read her nametag. She went on to say, "You must be here for breast cancer." That bunker in my chest was a dead giveaway. From somewhere in the depths of my navel, my voice was marshalling itself to be heard and eventually quietly acknowledged her observations. "Well, why don't you just come and sit right over here with us," she said. It was more a directive than a question. I picked up my toast and cheese and followed her to a table where I was introduced to a number of other "guests". As I assessed the group gathered around the table, I noted that everyone was about twenty years my senior, a fact that interested me. There seemed to be a lot of friendly ribbing jostling back and forth. A few of the men were teasing some of the women, with impish grins on their faces much as they must have looked at age ten in the schoolyard, minus the freckles, of course. It wasn't long at all before I was enjoying myself, caught up in getting to know the interesting faces gathered there. In retrospect, I was thankful to Phyllis, the lady who pulled me out of my shell and brought me into the warm, friendly support of the group. She had been a teacher, prior to retirement, and she seemed to know just what to do with my turtle shell and me.

The man across the table addressed a few of the others, asking: "How much longer do you have to go?" The responses came one after the other—one week, four weeks, seven weeks, and so on. "And what are you in for?" he asked me. "Breast cancer," I replied. The lady at the end of the table advised that she was there for cervical cancer, most of the fellas were there for prostate cancer, and a good many of the women announced that they were also there to be treated for breast cancer. Others announced colon cancer, lung cancer, and brain tumours. Phyllis had been to the Lodge four times previously, to accompany her husband during his treatment program. But this time, it was her turn for treatment. I understood without explanation that she was now a widow and noted with interest the evolution she must be feeling in her relationship with this kind and gentle place.

This was how we all began our acquaintance with each other. Over the next month or so, I would observe and participate in the cycles of newly formed friendships coming and going from the Lodge with the beginning and ending of each treatment program. Breast cancer people were usually there for five weeks and those with prostate cancer were there for seven weeks. Most other cases seemed to fall in and around those schedules. The queries of "What are you in for? How much longer do you have to go? When are you getting out?" amused me each time. We were not unlike a group of inmates in prison, and yet it was really only the query that was prison-like and not our surroundings. Most people looked quite healthy, zipping outside for their morning walk each day and returning for toast and coffee in the dining room with a healthy, glowing face. I could see that there was a possibility of feeling quite comfy here, as these seasoned people scooped me up and brought me into the fold.

My first true radiation treatment was to be at ten a.m. that Monday. I felt no apprehension as I made my way down the hall, and down the elevator to the radiation unit. I had been well trained. The dry run was to be exactly what I would experience once it came to the real thing, and that had proven to be quite uneventful. I swiped my health card into the computer system to signal my arrival to the radiation team and was ushered from the general waiting area to a smaller waiting room attached to LINAC2. There were three radiation machines in separate rooms, each identified by its name: LINAC1,

LINAC2 and LINAC3. A few minutes later, a radiation therapist came along to collect me and brought me into the inner sanctum of LINAC2.

The large room was papered in a dusty rose muted stripe; there were exceptional watercolour paintings every few feet. Andrea Bocelli's voice was singing Santa Lucia. I appreciated the music. It wasn't the usual piped-in elevator music but something special playing for the people in the radiation rooms. Soft fluorescent lighting ran around the perimeter of the room, creating a peaceful atmosphere similar to that of a fine dining restaurant. In the centre of the room was a significant piece of machinery that looked to be a huge overhanging arm stretching over the bed, on which I was to lie. There were four therapists in the room. I smiled to myself. One of the elderly ladies in the dining room had indignantly been convinced that the radiation therapists were not old enough to be out of school yet, and they had apparently assured her that they were really older than they looked—thirty-something would have been my guess.

One therapist held a pillowcase in front of my chest for privacy as I removed my sweatshirt. I appreciated the gesture to preserve my dignity. I would find this an amusing process by session #20, since once on the bed, the cloth is removed and the chest exposed for a team conference and numerous careful measurements. However, it was very helpful that first day, when I didn't yet know the team. I lay myself down on the bed and positioned my head and arms into the previously tailor-made alpha cradle. A massive piece of the radiation technology hung over my face, about a foot away, and looked no different to me than an X-ray machine. The therapists advised that they would be discussing the setup with each other and that I could just tune them out. If they needed my attention, they would address me by name. I was pleased to mentally slip into the role of observer.

It seemed that about fifteen minutes of discussion went on, lots more drawing on my chest, and affirmations of measures at "93.5" and "88 – 5" and "four-in-the-floor" called out to the other members of the team. They were very intent about getting it just right. The thought had occurred to me that I wouldn't like them to radiate my heart. I was relieved to see the scientific process transpiring and appreciated the competence that I felt emanating throughout every corner of the room. I didn't yet realize that this meticulous process would occur without fail each and every day that I would have a treatment.

The peripheral fluorescent lighting was snapped off. The room was in darkness except for the dimly lit amber pot lights shining directly above me. The light would come on in the radiation arm hanging directly above me. I could see a glow of a measurement gauge reflecting on my chest, as it was skilfully moved along until the precise contact point from above was made by the reflected "X" on my skin. My impressionable imagination watched what was possible from a horizontal position. The lighting was surreal. The vision of the therapists who were gathered around me, with their white lab coats glowing from the light of the radiation machine above, caused me to think in the darkness that this must be what it would be like to be abducted by aliens for medical experimentation and the harvesting of human reproductive seeds for heaven-only-knows-what. . . .

Activity in the room seemed to come to a standstill, and a therapist said softly to me, "Here we go." Then one by one they quickly disappeared behind the foot-thick protective wall, leaving me alone in the darkened room. My heart started to pound but I reminded myself that there was no need for concern. They had oriented me to the fact that they would be able to hear me at any time as they operated the computer that would activate my radiation. The dosage of radiation would be regulated by the computer system in the outer room; it was not possible to get an overdose. It stood to good reason that they wouldn't want to be in the room for the hundreds and hundreds of radiation patients with whom they would work over the years.

I saw the light on the wall change from green to yellow to red and prepared myself for RADIATION. A buzz emanated from the machine above me. It sounded like the lower buzz of a granddaddy bumblebee and then switched to a higher-pitched insolent mosquito. The buzzing continued for what seemed like a few minutes, then abruptly stopped and they were all back in the room with me. "What, no blue beam of light?" I thought. Nothing in the room had changed. I felt nothing at all. The arc of the radiation machine was shifted away with a mechanical motion, down to the bottom left of the table. Once again measurements were confirmed and there was a gentle announcement of "Here we go," and they were gone again. It reminded me of Oprah's musky voice cutting through the opening music of her program, announcing, "Here we go," just as her show is about to begin. The bumblebee and mosquito were back, this time a little longer. The arc of the machine was changed again to my right-hand side at about two o'clock from my perspective and then again over to the bottom left. There were four positions altogether. The radiation itself took only about five minutes all in all. The therapists returned, advising me that I could put my arms down, removing the pillow from below my knees and curling an elbow into mine to help me into a sitting position.

And so it went, each day for five weeks. I became very comfortable with the team of therapists in no time. I enjoyed their humour and admired their competence. One day as I entered the radiation room, I caught one therapist dancing away to the music. He was full of beans at the best of times, and seemed to want to lighten the atmosphere for everyone. He was successful! Another day, the session had concluded and an arm was offered to help raise me to a sitting position. I sat up but my wig remained on the alpha cradle. I could feel a split second hesitation at laughter in case my pride had been destroyed but once the therapist saw that I found it hilarious, she laughed along with me. These were people that I endearingly felt belonged to my cast of guardian angels. So professional, so precise, so patient, dealing with one person after another, all day, every day, week in and week out. I suspected that they worked very long hours. There is an extreme shortage of qualified radiation therapists, which likely magnifies their workload. They carry a huge responsibility in this massive quest to heal cancer.

Many people who arrived at the Lodge the following week were closer to my own age and some much younger. The range was from about twenty-seven to eighty-six years old. My roommate arrived the morning of my third day at the Lodge. She seemed a friendly sort. We chatted for a while and got to know one another, comparing our lumpectomies and mastectomies—the usual introductory conversation. She would be there for five weeks of radiation as well. We compared notes regarding personal comfort needs in sharing a room together. She wanted the room as cold as possible and I thought for certain I'd jump up and hug her. I just about never met anyone that liked a fresh cool room as much as I did, especially for sleeping. Once that was settled she went her own way much of the time and that left me with some space to be alone.

My new roomie was immediately scooped up by a group of women who enjoyed playing euchre until midnight each evening. So we traveled in different spheres throughout our stay, but connected often and enjoyed each other when we did. After the first night, I was greatly relieved to find out that we both snored with gusto! I relaxed, knowing that she wasn't going to put me out on the windowsill, charged with creating disruptions during the night. It seemed that we would get along well together.

Each week, we guests at the Daffodil Lodge had an appointment with our radiation oncologist in the treatment centre. It was a checkpoint for side effects and an opportunity for questions. Indeed! I had a question. I had been ruminating over it for some months. I had heard of a woman with thyroid cancer who was injected with a dye into her system to allow the radiation oncologist to see just where the cancer was and the progress in reducing it. I didn't know if this was actually possible, but was most curious about what had been termed a "massive invasion" of my lymph nodes and hoped the same could be done for me. I wanted to get confirmation when my treatment was finished, that the cancer had left my body completely. It was like getting to the end of a significant job and knowing that my mission had been accomplished. I wanted some closure. My doctor advised me that for the lymphatic system, this was not yet possible. I could see the concern in her face as she explained to me that research was currently being done in this area, but there was nothing ready for trial as yet.

I was actually quite despondent about that news for a day or two. It didn't seem fair that I would have to wonder and worry after all my hard work. But perpetuating a feeling of despondency is not something I have a talent for over an extended time frame. For me, it is like swimming to the bottom of the pool. I can stay down there for a short time, and then my body involuntarily floats back up to the surface in a rush of bubbles, seeking the sunshine. My rising from the depths was activated by a thought. It struck me that all the healthy people walking around in this world don't know when they are going to die either. To be counted on that side of the equation was much more preferable than to be on the other, with a confirmed death sentence. That point being well considered, I pulled up my pantyhose and moved on.

Social life at the Lodge was not to be sneezed at, I discovered. Events were planned and people were free to join in or abstain without any hint of cajoling. Our volunteer students organized a super Halloween party, complete with pumpkin carving and scavenger hunts throughout the Lodge. Most of the guests brought costumes from home, dressed up and had a blast. It was the talk of the town throughout the entire treatment facility the following day. A shopping trip was coordinated one evening, with a van of enthusiastic "shop-till-you-drop" types, gathering for dinner at East Side Mario's for sustenance before hitting the local mall. I showed up for bingo one night and actually had a good time. There was shuffleboard, and teams for terribly complicated jig saw puzzles, and great movie nights, popcorn and all. We were entertained one fine evening by the Air Force 22 Wing Band coming from the air base in my hometown. Nick, one of our own from the Lodge, was part of the band. He delighted in taking up his usual position with the brass, to play for us on the last night of his seven-week treatment program. He was grinning from ear to ear.

A close friend invited me to her home for dinner once a week during my stay in her city. It was a welcome diversion. Sandra is a fabulous cook and lots of fun. It was no wonder that I would awaken in the morning, brightened by the prospect of a visit with her that evening. And then there was the day that Bruce came to town mid-week and surprised me. I was elated to see him. He took me for a delicious long browse around my favourite bookstore and then out for a beautiful Italian dinner that evening. We stayed at a local motel, in a lovely room with a king-size bed and wonderful pillows. . . . Not to worry. I was on time for my radiation appointment the next day.

The dining room at the Lodge was an excellent perch for people-watching. I noted an interesting phenomenon in our genders. In the morning, when it was time for coffee and toast, the female population gathered mainly around a large rectangular table, generating waves of laughing chatter. An incoming participant replaced each departing female in the circle, as people disappeared to attend their radiation or chemo appointments. On the other hand, the male guests would come in to the dining room, greet everyone in a chipper manner and proceed with their breakfast to one of the round tables where they could be alone, to look out the window at the awakening morning, and get their thinking done for the day. It seemed to be the inherent "lone wolf" in them. Later in the day, they would sometimes cluster a little more in groups; and definitely in the evening, in the TV rooms designated sports only, where we would find enthusiastic groups of gentlemen enjoying "the game" and each other's company.

There were people from all walks of life and fascinating circumstances. There were the two friends from a smaller northern community, Georgina and Janine. Georgina baked exceptional butter tarts for all of us; Janine always affectionately called me "Schnooks" and I loved them both. They had grown up together, gone all through school together and now, as a matter of coincidence, here they were somewhere in their sixties, sharing a room together, as well as an experience with breast cancer. There was the math professor, who looked to be in his early fifties, well conditioned and looking healthy enough to compete in a triathlon. It turned out that he was a very close friend of a previous boss of mine. I was floored when he told me they had discovered his prostate cancer in the most serious stage, a level ten. It was evident to me that he would have been meticulous about his health all his life. We were avid researchers by nature and we compared and swapped books about cancer in an effort to share the knowledge. There were two women whose sisters were also being treated for breast cancer at different medical facilities at the same time as they were undergoing radiation and chemotherapy. That statistic of one in every eight women being diagnosed with breast cancer this year is staggering in and of itself, let alone to think of two sets of sisters from different families experiencing breast cancer at the same time.

Gwen was the tiniest, spunkiest, women I had ever met in my entire life. Her eyes were a brilliant sapphire blue, and her snow-white hair framed a face full of mischief and energy. Every morning she had her little sneakers on and went for a power walk for miles around the adjacent lake. She stayed up until midnight every night playing euchre, and always had enough spark to be a delightful part of the group. The fact that she was seventy-six years of age simply amazed me. I wished to myself that I would be that alive and on fire when I reach that age, and then I reminded myself that I didn't feel that full of energy when I was twenty-six, let alone seventy-six. Abundant, sustained Energy! That would be on my new list of priorities when all this was over.

One of my new friends told us a story one morning at coffee around the dining room table. I admired a golden brooch of a cow that she was wearing on her blouse. She smiled in a rather secretive way and said, "Well, you know, there is a real story to this brooch.

"A number of years ago, when I was shopping with my daughters, I saw a brooch just like this in the jewelry counter of a store, but it was pewter. The girls thought it a silly purchase, but I wanted it and so I bought it. For some reason, it appealed to me.

"One night, I went out for dinner alone. [I wasn't sure if she was a widow or a divorcee, but didn't like to ask.] When I stepped into the dining room, the maitre-de greeted me. Looking at a gentleman who had come in behind me from the parking lot, the maitre-de picked up his menus and inquired, 'For two?' I told him that I was alone, but unfortunately he only had a table for two. The gentleman beside me asked if I minded if we shared the table.

"I was hesitant, but I agreed, not wanting to see him go without dinner. It was a very interesting conversation throughout the evening. He must have been a little nervous because he took a drink from the carafe of wine by mistake, but I just pretended that I hadn't noticed. The party at the table next to us noticed, however. I was wearing my pewter cow brooch. He admired it and to my surprise informed me that he was a cattle rancher."

Then our storyteller looked coyly down at her cup of coffee, smiled a mischievous smile, looked up again at us and said confidentially, "And we've been together ever since." The man that became her new husband borrowed the pewter cow brooch from her, had the pattern copied and had one made specially for her in gold.

I was completely enchanted by this story. I sat back in my chair and looked around at all the special faces and the company I was enjoying. I thought to myself, "The secret is out. The Daffodil Terrace Lodge is neither depressing nor boring. It's actually a very special place."

A new young woman had joined us in the dining room. She stood apart from everyone else, looking lost and alone. I could see big tears rolling down her cheeks as she stood quietly looking down at the floor. It seemed time for me to extend the welcome that I was once given, shelter her with my wing and bring her into the nest. I would do this on a number of occasions when lost souls arrived. During my last week at the Lodge, I noticed that these people in turn would step forward to take their place in the welcoming committee, just as Phyllis had taught me through her example. It was an unspoken rite of passage as the cycles of people continued to arrive and leave, and new friendships were formed.

We drove away from the Daffodil Terrace Lodge on my last day, all the good-bye's having been said. The hugs were laden with good wishes. I was thrilled to be going home but sad to be leaving my new friends. The highway was washed in sunshine on this wonderful November morning. Even the weeds in the ditch along the highway took on a new presence where summer's sunshine had roasted their hues. The foot of the rock cuts lining the highway were laced with cattails, tall shafts of wheat, dried Queen Anne's lace and rusted ferns. The water in the lakes had turned to a cold slate gray. My latent artistic talent longed to paint the rich stands of maple, birch and bright golden tamarack in their full glory. A flock of geese flew over our heads, heading south for the winter. They flew in perfect V formation, supporting each other, taking turns at the lead when necessary, knowing instinctively the needs of the rest of the flock. I thought of my friends at the Lodge. Every now and again, people in a group are exposed to a momentous experience that will change their lives forever. We often see this during wartime. Through this experience, I felt the bond of a group of people who had been shipwrecked on an island together. We shared our "rations" and boosted each other when spirits weakened. We formed deep relationships, some of which will continue on. Regardless, I know these acquaintances will be held dear in our memories. I closed my eyes to envision the faces around the dining room table and etched them into my memory for all time. I will think of them often. That way they'll always be with me.

Chapter 11

The Spouse Speaks

Dear Reader,

As the spouse of a cancer patient, I know many others will share my journey. When I first learned about Pat's illness, nowhere was I able to find a resource that gave me an insider's look at the partner's role. As that well known cliché states, "If I knew then what I know now, I could have been better prepared [for this crisis]." I hope the following narrative helps to fill that gap for some of you.

To write, or not to write, that has been the question for me for some time now.

So why my reluctance—was it the male ego? Perhaps I felt this was Pat's book. My involvement was really insignificant compared to what she went through. Did I really want to relive this experience? Was I ready to share some rather personal thoughts? An attempt to give a unique perspective to assist other spouses, partners, family and friends was part of the inner motivation that helped me to leap the hurdle of reluctance. In the long run this would also assist the patient, and that's truly most important.

There's no doubt that upon hearing from your spouse or partner the words, "I feel a lump in my breast," you will feel as though a two-by-four has been swung in a wide arc landing right on your chest. This can be the beginning of a long road never before travelled.

As each medical step is taken with the anticipation of hearing good news (or bad), the build up of tension begins to take its toll, usually not noticed by you at the time. Generally, the worry is with the primary patient and recognizing the anxiety she must be experiencing. She is the one who will be directly affected as each stage unfolds. It's her body, her breast, her mortality. Believe me, she is not alone in this journey, nor does she want to be. You are her partner in the truest sense of the word, so give her the signal verbally, or by actions as men tend to do, that you are with her and will experience what life unfolds as if joined at the hip. As a spouse, you are in for a turbulent ride as well. I now fully understand when so many people asked me, "So, how are you doing?" "How are *you* coping?" "It must be difficult?" At the time those questions just didn't seem to fit the scenario, since after all it was Pat who had cancer. I now know otherwise.

We were told that surgery would be exploratory and if things did not look good, removal of her breast would be necessary. This is the first of at least two occasions that your partner will need the utmost assurance that no matter what the result, you will love her and you both will adjust to the outcome together. The second occasion is if indeed a mastectomy occurs. Make no mistake about it, there is a period of adjustment, for both of you.

One of the most difficult days was "surgery day." I suppose my anxiety stemmed from my personal feeling of helplessness with no control over the situation whatsoever. After I accompanied Pat through the checking-in processes, the nurses indicated that the operation would take an hour or two and there was a "quiet room" on the floor if I wished to stay there. I knew I would eventually park myself there, but not right away. My head and my body were spinning with emotions when Pat was wheeled away from me and into the operating room. I was completely powerless. It was a case of waiting for the news, with Pat somewhere in the depths of the hospital. An hour or two!

I decided to leave the hospital for a half hour, drive Woody to a favourite spot on the shore of our city's wonderful lake, and try to deal with my emotions. They ran the gamut, from as upbeat as possible, hoping that the exploratory surgery would reveal a benign lump, no problem, to a great fear of what the surgeon would find and the effect on Pat's future. During that period at the lake I was able to sort myself out and although I knew I was really keyed up, at the same time a realistic, calm determination came over me to accept and handle whatever the day brought. I returned to the quiet room to take up my vigil, which lasted close to three hours. So much went through my thoughts as the minutes, then hours, ticked by.

Finally the surgeon arrived. Looking me in the eye, she stated that the surgery went very well, but an invasion of the lymph nodes appeared to have occurred. Pat's future treatments would include chemotherapy, radiation, and taking Tamoxifen for approximately five years. Up to this point, I was trying to grasp the news and its implications. The doctor didn't mention whether or not the breast (or breasts) was removed. So I asked. "Yes" was the response. One breast was removed.

Well, this was the beginning of a whole new world that many individuals do not have knowledge of—the medical treatment of cancer patients. Yes, everyone knows of the disease. They have heard of the treatments—chemotherapy and radiation. They have heard of the side effects. Unless someone has been personally involved, however, the whole process is somewhat of a mystery. I'm not sure if it's because I'm now intimately acquainted with this disease, but it seems only recently that cancer patients, particularly those with "celebrity" status, have stepped into the public eye with their hats, wigs, scarves, and bare heads to speak of their journey. This mystery surrounding cancer and its treatment makes it incumbent on the patient and family to use whatever resources are available, including first-hand account books, such as this one, videos, etc. The resource material is quite abundant and excellent. Much of the information is in pamphlet form, making the absorption of this new knowledge much easier. This is certainly one method of gaining some control of one's destiny, as well as becoming a full participant in the treatment.

I can tell you that the partner's role is an unknown factor at the beginning of the treatment. In hindsight, I didn't expect the caregiver's role to be such a major one, but it can be. I recognize that some individuals are not inclined to be as involved directly as I was. In this instance, I'm speaking of changing bandages, applying soothing lotions, temperature-taking, placing cool cloths on the patient's forehead, and giving a steadying arm for support to walk what may be only a few steps. The other peripheral role expands one hundred percent, to meal preparation, cleaning, dishes, grocery shopping, and so on.

Then we have the patient's schedule of medical appointments and treatments, which in our case meant three hours' return travel time to the cancer centre for chemotherapy every second week, with trips to the local hospital during the alternate weeks. All radiation treatments were done at the cancer centre, which involved weekly trips as well. So there you have it in a nutshell. Now don't be discouraged by all this activity; most of it occurs in a natural fashion, and there is "down time" for you. That's your opportunity to continue on with your hobbies, sports, walking the dog, whatever your normal routine would be. I believe your spouse expects and wishes you to continue to be involved in your other interests.

Is there a piece missing for you? What about my job, you ask? Well fortunately, I'm retired. Of course that springs a lot of time, doesn't it? Yet on the other hand it doesn't. You folks who are retired will know what I mean.

In any case, I'm sure that continuing to work wouldn't exclude the employed spouse from taking on whatever was possible. I would stress here that it is extremely important for the spouse to negotiate as much leave time as possible from work so that he can provide maximum patient support. You can be certain that vacation time will not be used in the true sense of the word for the next six to twelve months at least, so there's a block of time that may be available. Many employers have discretionary leave available for critical times such as this. In addition, the work-from-home alternative at crucial times could prove quite acceptable to both employer and employee. Although not every day is swallowed up by patient support, on those days where medical appointments are required there's a one- to two-hour window where leave from employment would be necessary. The alternative, of course, is to take up the many offers of help from family and friends. Likewise, there are the community support, homecare and homemaker programs available. For example, the Cancer Society has a "patient-ride" program to take people to their treatment appointments. In addition, the Society can provide or refer patients to a multitude of other support services. The bottom line is, the comfort you can help create for the patient pays you back with a sense of helping in the recovery process, and that is priceless.

Humour is another key in adjusting to what would appear as a rather serious situation. For example, one day shortly after Pat's surgery when she was confined to bed, I decided to place a dinner bell on her nightstand. This was a sentimental item of Pat's that we usually put out on display as part of our Christmas decorations. Our master bedroom is on the second floor of our home and I was concerned that I might not hear Pat calling. I could tell that the bell idea was not going over too big with Pat, and I surmised that to "summon me" would be the last thing she would want to do. I had assumed that if she were ill and required help, it would be an excellent way to get my attention, as indeed she was quite weak. So we both sort of smiled at this idea of mine and off I went back down the stairs to settle down to some reading. I had it in the back of my mind that the situation would be very serious before Pat would ring that bell.

Approximately fifteen minutes later I heard a faint melodic tinkle. Well, out of my chair I sprang, and thundered up the stairs three at a time. As I approached the bedroom door I heard Pat saying to me, "No, no, there's nothing wrong!" Her intent was to try out this method of communication and see how it worked. She expected me to respond verbally so that she could say to me, "The next time you come upstairs would you bring up a . . .?" We had a good chuckle and Pat used the bell on further occasions when my reaction was much more casual. One thing that experience did point out to me, though, was that my "adrenalin button" was on high, ready for the next crisis. I had not realized my own state of tension and anticipation.

Speaking of adrenaline, another story comes to mind. Pat and I tried to create an atmosphere of normalcy, which included outings such as walks or drives, or enjoying an ice cream cone. However, a startling event on a beautiful fall afternoon certainly tested us. We were winding down a wonderful Thanksgiving weekend. We had invited our family over for Thanksgiving dinner and enjoyed a great visit with my long-lost cousin Penny, who is like a sister I never had. Pat and I were able to pull off the turkey dinner and visit with what we believed was a success and a good feeling of accomplishment. (We initially had thought neither of us was up to it.) The chemotherapy sessions were over at long last, with radiation treatments to commence within a week. Walks of any length were not feasible for Pat as yet, so a casual drive through some of our favourite residential neighborhoods sure seemed in order. Off we went. Woody was in the back seat with his head out the window enjoying whatever dogs get out of this. Up the streets, down the streets, around the corners; nothing like a slow drive to relax and enjoy life. The fall afternoon was beautiful, sunny, warm, and vibrant with colour.

Suddenly it was as though someone had snapped his fingers to change the scene. We went from total enjoyment and serenity, to dealing with a shrieking, yelping dog with his head caught in the power window. Woody had inadvertently stepped on the power button on the armrest. Up went the window, catching his throat and jamming his head outside. His front paws were flailing frantically on the power button, which continued to jam the window tighter and tighter on his throat. Can you picture it? Can you feel it? For some unknown reason the driver's master control buttons wouldn't work. Stopping the car, we both jumped out, trying to pull the window down manually. Pat was close to hysteria, trying with all her might to hold the window down. I'm trying to work Woody's head back through the window with no luck. The gap was just too small. Then back into the car, trying the power buttons once again . . . nothing! A passing jogger attempts to assist us. Woody's eyes are bulging in terror. His saliva is foaming at the edges of his mouth. Breaking the window seems the only solution. I search in the trunk, can't find the tire iron fast enough. Pat is crying and screaming, pulling at the window with all her strength to stop it from strangling the dog. I have a golf club in my hand. Could the dog's throat be cut if I smash the window? Back to the power button, which works, finally! What a sense of relief! It took hours to recover from that episode. The shock numbed us for the rest of the weekend and even to this day we get shivers just thinking about it.

There are three morals to this Woody's Window story. The first, no matter what atmosphere you try to create, destiny can sure take some unexpected twists. Second, the body is some mysterious creation, considering Pat's weakened condition and the strength she produced when the mind/body phenomenon kicked into gear.

Third, always ensure the driver's lock is engaged on the power windows!

A couple of other hints in dealing with the adjustment period come to mind. Perhaps the greatest and most sensitive adjustment is to the fact of your partner losing her breast or, in some cases, breasts. She, of course, will be the most sensitive about this new situation and will no doubt feel very awkward. She will go out of her way to make sure you do not catch sight of the battleground on her chest. You will need to respect her feelings and I can tell you that as she gets used to this change in her body, time will ease her awkwardness. Believe it or not, you both will accept what has happened. It's not difficult to remember that this surgery saved her life.

An instance that calls for adjustment and sensitivity on your part is the onset of your partner's hair loss. Quite likely the first signs will be clumps of hair just coming out by the handful. In many cases, as in Pat's, head baldness is not the only symptom, but elsewhere as well, including eyebrows and eyelashes that take a beating from chemotherapy treatments. As I understand it, hair loss is dependent on the type and strength of chemotherapy. So if there's an aggressive chemo treatment planned, hair loss is inevitable. The good news is that the hair does grow back, beginning shortly after chemo treatments stop. Another key to the patient's self-consciousness and self-esteem is the head covering, whatever that may be. A wig is no doubt in order. This is no time to save pennies, as only the better wigs are a convincing replacement for the real thing. This doesn't always mean an outlay of a lot of money, as in some cases wigs are available, free, at some treatment centers. Otherwise, most health plans cover this item. You can sure help her decide on the most suitable style and this can turn into quite the project. Her "new hair" could be hers for a year or so. Don't be surprised if she ends up with a different style and/or a different colour than usual.

Discouragement leading to mild or severe depression can set in rather often with cancer patients. Be on the alert for this sign and do your best to offer encouragement, listen, change the scenery, tip off the visiting nurse (if there is one), or get a professional counsellor to step in.

I have a great respect for the drugs used in chemotherapy. They are life-giving, while also very powerful and toxic. Confidentially, between you and me, should you be kissing your mate (and you should be) don't be surprised if she tastes different. I can only describe it as a metallic taste. Let me assure you that the taste disappears when chemo treatment ends.

Although this journey is certainly not one anyone would take by choice, there are bound to be some unexpected benefits as a result. Some of the changes that may occur are a healthier lifestyle, a renewal of closeness and appreciation for each other, and an enhanced understanding of what's really important in life. I can tell you that my observation of life from the perspective of the "cancer world" has had a great impact on me. One of the most poignant experiences was my first visit to the chemotherapy unit, where people from young children, to adolescents, to adults both young and elderly, were in their large recliner chairs or stretched out on beds, receiving chemotherapy treatments intravenously. There were at least fifteen to twenty individuals at any given time, with the faces changing about every two hours. This apparently goes on every weekday. At that moment I made a pact with myself that I would stop smoking. Approximately six months later I had my last cigarette. As I write this, I have been smoke-free for eight months, with absolutely no intention of returning to that habit.

I'm about to close this chapter, and I'll summarize some of the key points that you might find helpful.

- Adjust to the news of cancer, side effects, life changes, together.
- There is no harm in exercising a sense of humour; in fact it brings a lot of good.
- Be honest with one another, and with the rest of the family and friends. People need this from you and it takes less effort.
- Both of you need to get out for a walk, even just a few steps if that's all your partner can do; but particularly drives—they're very therapeutic.
- Take time for yourself.
- The patient needs rest, and so will you.
- Don't be surprised when, after your partner's treatment ends, and life just begins to get back to normal, the impact hits you.

That's when you realize the stress you've been under. To know this at the beginning of the journey and take appropriate measures as you go along, will assist.

- My last suggestion is for both of you to plan a reward for each other when the journey is over, such as a special vacation. This may take some fancy planning economically, but the key is to plan for it.

Safe journey,

Bruce

Chapter 12

On Being Positive

Sometimes life can be like boring a hole through a mountain with a feather duster.

When you have cancer, everyone says, "Just be positive." There are a lot of dimensions to be considered in this business of "being positive." When I was in high school, my principal called me down to his office one day. It seemed that I had failed math again. I was capable of more and he felt that a chat was in order. "Patsy," he said—I always hated being called Patsy—"you are an incurable optimist and you're never going to get anywhere!" It was one of those so-called "wisdoms" that one holds in one's memory bank for a lifetime. I have gone through a number of earth-shattering losses in my years. I often think of that silly statement and mentally explain to that man in my most cool, calm, superior adult voice, that I have done quite well for myself, thank you very much, and had it not been for my eternal optimism I would have thrown in the towel some twenty years ago. And another thing, there is life after grade eleven math!

I would be the first to agree that a positive outlook is essential to living and to dealing with cancer. However, if you have been diagnosed with cancer, we should talk.

There is a time and a place for being positive and it's significantly important to understand the distinction. When those around you become aware of your cancer, you will definitely hear the advice, "BE POSITIVE" over and over again. I think that people say this because they want to help and they don't know what else to do; and they don't realize that there is a period where this advice is not all that helpful. We have to remember that it can sometimes be more difficult to be the bystander to a loved one with cancer than it is to actually be the cancer patient. When others say this to us, they hope to keep us safe and well. But you can't spare someone's feelings by denying them. We need to understand that the strength of being positive comes from within. It is an intrinsic frame of mind and not something that can be cast upon someone from an external source, like some sort of magic spell.

One of my cousins who survived breast cancer wrote a very good article for the *Toronto Star*, a national newspaper, some years ago. Here is some of her insight on being positive that will be helpful to those with cancer and those who support them:

> With the prevalence of women experiencing breast cancer, I feel the need to address each of their friends and loved ones who would like to know how to support them.

> Keep in mind, having been diagnosed with breast cancer and suddenly undergoing a mastectomy and/or other treatments, a woman is overwhelmed with her new world of uncertainties and is grieving her losses.

> In her book, *The Breast Cancer Companion* (William Morrow and Company Ltd., 1993) Kathy LaTour, a breast cancer survivor, explains the grief and lists the possible losses:

> Loss of health, loss of body part, loss of femininity/feeling of being attractive, loss of self-concept that we are healthy, loss of significant relationship, of innocence, of guarantee of the future, of family as we knew it, of the chance to bear a child, financial stability, job, control over life, loss of the persons we used to be, goals and dreams, loss of significant other, of ability to fill the parental role. Thus a woman must grieve.

> To those who are concerned, support your friend or loved one by acknowledging the fears and anxieties. "It will never be over for the rest of my life because I'll always worry it's going to come back," states one of the women LaTour interviewed.

> To the significant other, assure her that she is still loved and is the same person.

Being a breast cancer survivor myself, it is my opinion that she cannot respond to the advice "Be positive." Rather, allow her to deal with her losses and her various emotions, and her attitude will take care of itself. "You can be positive and still accept the fact that you are angry and afraid," LaTour writes.

My cousin, whose name is Marjorie Urquhart, closes her article by saying, "I would like others to receive the understanding and caring that I am given; it aids in healing."

I would like to add my own two cents to Marjorie's words. For those friends and family members who want to connect with someone who has been diagnosed with cancer, it can be difficult to know what to say. I experienced this bystander's view when both my mother and my father had cancer. My father seemed to slip into a six-month oblivion of sadness and non-communication between his diagnosis and his death. I wanted so very badly to connect with him but was never successful in finding the right words to open that doorway. What a loss for both of us. Later there were also people with whom I worked going through cancer. For those who were not family, it was easier to avoid the person and hope that my prayers and my caring from afar would in some way be helpful. I didn't want to say something that would make matters worse and I just didn't have any magic words to make it better. But now that I have walked in the slippers of the cancer patient, I *do* know what to say and perhaps it will help others. It's very simple:

"I was sorry to hear that you have cancer. How are you coping?"

The trick is then to be silent and be a good listener. It's an open-ended question that prevents a curt answer of "yes" or "no," as would happen if you changed the wording ever so slightly to say, "Are you coping all right?" With this question, depending on the individual, an opportunity to open up a lot of bottled thoughts and feelings might be missed. You don't need to say, "Be positive." If the person is at the point where she can have a good outlook, she'll be happy to tell you all about it. If you worry about showing your own emotion, don't give it another thought. It won't offend the person to know that you care.

For those who have just been diagnosed with cancer, there is a bridge that you must cross along this journey. You can't hop over it, slither under it, or tippy-toe around it. I told you about the tunnel at the beginning of this journey, and the chilly and lonely moonlit field along the way. Before you come to the mountain, you must cross the bridge. It's a rope bridge made from long, fibrous vines. It will sag with your weight and sway in the wind. The vines are strong and truly will hold you. Some people panic like a deer in the headlights, and they sit down halfway across, frozen with fear and unable to move on.

But here is something you need to think about. Many have crossed this bridge before you. The more of us that cross over, the stronger the bridge becomes. It's the faith and the hope of every person taking this challenge that strengthens those vines. Once you become deeply angry at this interruption to your life, your safety and your happiness, it's time to cry. With each of these steps, you put one foot in front of the other. You may get angry again, and cry again. There is no limit to the number of times you might repeat these footsteps. It's a very individual thing. When you are crossing the bridge, don't look down and don't look across. Just concentrate on each step—never mind the panoramic view. It's too big to take in all at one time.

Think back to the healing cycle I shared with you. At this point, the one step in the cycle that I would recommend you spend as little time in as possible is Denial. It will hold you back, delaying your journey. Get educated. Get angry. Talk it over with a friend or someone who is a good listener. Cry. Be sad. Talk it out again. If you are having trouble accessing those emotions, I'll share with you a sure-fire way to uncork the bottle. Update your will (which you should do anyway) and write a letter to each person that is dear to you. Leave the letters tucked safely away with your will. You don't need to mention them to anyone. Tell the people close to you what you would want them to know if anything should ever happen to you. Tell them about the wishes and the hopes that you have for them and what they have meant to you. I guarantee that you won't get through this exercise without a clearing of emotion. Will it be bad for your state of mind? I think not. It's a reality that we all must face and whether we are going to go now or thirty years from now, the fact of the matter is that we will all leave this world someday—and this from an eternal optimist. So, I say again, allow yourself to be angry, to feel the fear, to be sad and to cry. And *then* you can safely and effectively move on to "BEING POSITIVE." Trying to bypass the discomfort of this phase will more likely leave you indefinitely in the clasp of Denial.

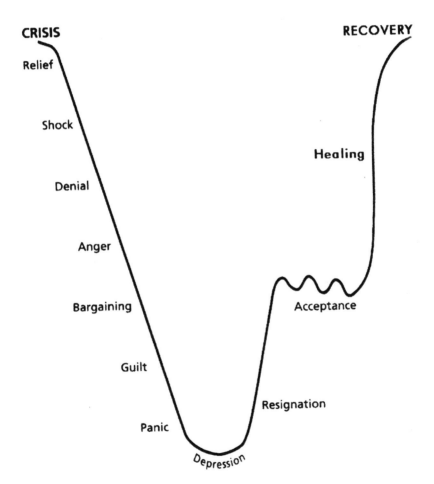

Modified and reproduced by special permission of the Publisher, Consulting Psychologists Press, Inc., Palo Alto, CA 94303 from **Type and Change MBTI®** **Leader's Guide,** by Nancy J. Barger and Linda K. Kirby. Copyright 1997 by Consulting Psychologists Press Inc. All rights reserved. Further reproduction is prohibited without the Publisher's written consent.

Depression is another step that one must take. And that's all right too. Just watch that you don't get stuck there. If you sense that you are not pulling out of it, go and talk to a professional. I had an interesting and helpful few sessions with an excellent counsellor in the Psychosocial Department of the medical centre where I received my treatment. I avoided that department as a resource for a long time, for some reason. Probably because unconsciously I didn't want to really look at all the things that were worrying me. Those thoughts were like a slow leaking valve that I had to gauge carefully and open only a bit at a time, when I was ready. The fact of the matter is that life goes on and so do its problems.

I was deeply concerned about losing my job through all the restructuring and downsizing my company was going through, and all the while I was trying to deal with this issue of cancer. I knew my employer could not legally dismiss me while I was on sick leave, but I also knew that it could happen to me, like anyone else, when I returned to work. I was obsessing over family finances and how to plan for the future and the present while on disability pay. I was worrying that my cancer would recur somewhere down the road, thrusting me back into treatment and again into the reduction of disability pay.

The worries started to get the best of me. My eternal optimism left me, as though my shadow had been severed. For several weeks I seemed to be "stuck" on the dark side of everything. My treatment program was coming to an end. I should have been elated about that, but instead I found myself despondent about having to leave this protective cocoon that I was in. I knew that in a few short weeks, the bubble would burst and I would be thrust back into that program called LIFE. I could feel the stress building to unmanageable proportions.

When I finally had the wisdom to exercise my resources, the social worker and I spent some time talking about problem-solving techniques. My overturned wagon was quickly set back on its wheels. I learned that in spite of using effective relaxation techniques, and thinking positively, these methods were no replacement for actually finding resolutions to my problems. They were only helping me to cope in the meantime. I have used problem-solving processes in business settings, but somehow, when the problem was this personal and this overwhelming, it was difficult to look at things objectively. Additionally, I had somehow merged many smaller problems together in my mind, making resolution seem like an insurmountable task. I needed someone to guide me. It helped a great deal for me to sit down with a pencil and paper to write all this out. The tried-and-true technique that I would like to recommend is as follows:

1. Accurately identify the problem. Be specific: How, What, When, Where, With Whom? Note if you have more than one problem clustered together; deal with each component as a completely separate process.

2. What would a resolution look like?

3. Generate alternatives. What are the possibilities? Quantity is the objective at this stage, not quality. Do not censor any ideas.

4. Evaluate the alternatives. What are the likely consequences of each alternative, both positive and negative?

5. Which of the above is most likely to be effective?

6. Is the solution chosen actually going to produce the desired outcome? If not, go back to Step #3.

7. What are the steps, the skills and the resources needed to work through the solutions? Who can help you with information?

8. Follow through on the action of your decision and observe whether or not your goal has indeed been achieved.

Here are some good reasons for "being positive," from an eternal optimist. With the occurrence of cancer at epidemic proportions, chances are that family members and friends are now, or about to, walk this same path someday in the future. I would want to create a low to non-existent terror factor for them. If my stepdaughter, my son-in-law or my sons were to go through this challenge, I would want them to think of my experience, the way that I have thought back to my mother's, and know that it really can be done and it doesn't have to mean the end of the world. I had many opportunities to make people suffer along with me, if I had chosen to give that profile to my experience. But what would that really have accomplished? We cancer patients have a responsibility to model the way, *but only after we ourselves have grieved.* I am not suggesting that we each require the competencies of Joan of Arc to do the job.

Being positive is an effective tool to visualizing yourself to wellness. Remember the mind-body connection and the influence your thoughts can have on your health. It is a well-known fact that stress worsens cancer and that lowering stress can lessen the deadly impact. I remind you again that you can't deal with stress until you release the negativity in your mind. Rather than terming this as "negative thinking," one should think of it as "de-stressing."

I recall a memory from many years ago of driving along in the car with one of my boys in the front seat beside me. Jordan was just a little fellow of five years. He had been quiet and in deep thought for some time, and suddenly let out a significantly long and audible sigh. I asked him what was wrong, and he responded so naturally and calmly saying, "Oh nothing, Mommy. I'm just letting all my air out."

That's what de-stressing is all about. It's like letting all the air out of an over-inflated beach ball. When you are de-stressing and when you are feeling positive and tapping your sense of humour, your immune system responds. Your immune system is your chief ally in the work that you will have to do throughout your treatment program. Give it the right environment. Feed it properly, give it lots of rest and fresh air and make it comfortable. You do have control over your outlook. It's a matter of choice, when the time is right.

I want to tell you about the very best resource that I uncovered. The book is called *Return to Wholeness: Embracing Body, Mind and Spirit in the Face of Cancer* by David Simon, M.D., who is the Medical Director for the Chopra Center for Well Being. It was published in 1999, and I found it to be artfully written, a knowledgeable and compassionate support that was very instrumental in helping me through the steps of my journey. Dr. Simon covers valuable material for those who have been diagnosed with any kind of cancer. He values the approach of both western and eastern medical practices.

The book covers many dimensions of the journey, as I have outlined here:

- Understanding cancer
- The immune system, impacts of stress and how to increase our immunity
- Nutritional healing—food as medicine
- Vitamins, minerals and other healing substances
- Herbs in cancer care
- The modern medical arsenal—chemotherapy, radiation, etc.
- Meditation and visualization
- Sensual nourishment and healing through sound, touch, sight and smell
- Harmonizing to the rhythm of nature
- Healing through expression—art therapy and journalling
- The science of humour
- Assessing and utilizing alternative medicine
- Approaching common cancers from the mind-body perspective
- Facing our fear of death by embracing life

A phrase that is repeated often throughout this book is in regard to establishing a commitment to wholeness: *"Our bodies are the end products of our experiences and interpretations. To change our bodies, we need to change our experiences. Make a commitment to change your life in the direction of greater love and caring for yourself and those close to you."* I read these words over and over again at the end of every chapter. Each chapter then offered the advice and guidance from a myriad of different perspectives that were not only leading me to the best circumstances for healing but also for a better way of living the rest of my life. I will read this book again and again.

The healing cycle has a positive milestone—an oasis along the journey. It is ACCEPTANCE. There is a timeworn saying, "When life gives you lemons, make lemonade." I think back to my stay at the Daffodil Terrace Lodge and the day I almost died in a fit of giggles. I talked for a long time with a man in the dining room one afternoon.

His name was Don, and I'll never forget him. He had my father's eyes and eyelashes. Eyes are so distinctly individual. I am not talking about the similar shape and colour that family members share. I am talking about the very essence of a spirit that the eyes carry to each soul and personality. One would think it impossible to duplicate from one person to another. And yet, here was this man with my father's eyes. He had a few teeth missing, not like my father. He wore a baseball cap, not like my father. But he very definitely had my father's eyes. He talked to me for a long time about his new satellite dish. He was intrigued with how it worked, all the features it carried and just what today's technology could accomplish.

Then, out of the blue he said, "Let me tell you about the day I lost my ass." And he began to tell me about his colostomy, resulting from colon cancer. I've told you before that I hate to hear the details of another person's physical pain, especially surgery. A squeaky little voice inside my head was shrieking, "Oh no, don't tell me all the gory details." But I remained outwardly calm and nodded my head to be a good listener. After all, we were all in this together. A few of us had gathered at the table by this point. He told us about the day he received the news, the words his doctor had said to him when he explained the extent of the proposed surgery that would change his life, and his gentle acceptance of the outcome. I thought I detected some sadness to his voice. But then his blue eyes twinkled, and he said, "So now if you want to kick me in the ass, you'll have to find it first." And he pointed to the front of his abdomen, where we assumed he was wearing a new colostomy bag. "I don't have to bother taking time to have a poop any more," he said, "and if anyone calls me an asshole, I know they're only referring to a plastic ring that fits with my new gizmo!" He was laughing and we were in stitches right along with him. He needed to tell that story to someone and along with it one could see that he was finding acceptance.

Sometimes my sense of humour, my sense of logic and/or my sense of the ridiculous would muster up new perspectives on things. My mother says that we share a sense of the ridiculous and that is the bond that glues us together. She is likely right. Turning negatives to positives can be like the metamorphosis of a caterpillar to a butterfly. I know my counsellor, Bertrand, would call it "reframing."

When my hair was all gone, I accepted it and welcomed the saving of $70.00 each month for professional hair maintenance. I didn't have to spend fifteen minutes each morning with the curling iron and my bottle of mousse, tediously trying to make every day a good hair day. And the added bonus was that I didn't have to shave my legs. Now we're talking pluses!

My chemotherapy medication cost a whopping $350.00 per month. I used my VISA Gold card to cover the costs each month, submitted my receipts for reimbursement to my insurance carrier, and accumulated travel points at the same time for a nice holiday somewhere in the future.

In temporarily leaving the job that I loved so much, the one I was stuck to like a suction cup, I discovered so many special things. I had the opportunity to stop and smell the purple coneflowers. I became reacquainted with my sons and enjoyed the involvement of helping to plan for their post secondary education. I had to learn how to talk with them as adults. I hadn't realized my interaction with them was stuck back at around age twelve. Time had passed me by. I had some very treasured time with my husband. His early retirement allowed us the luxury of spending days and weeks together, talking, walking, enjoying a good bowl of soup in a cozy restaurant and sitting silently with one another, something my fast-paced professional life had excluded almost entirely. I found my soul, my inner being, and I can't adequately explain the peace this has brought to me. As a result, all components of my life seem to have shifted into a much better perspective.

I discovered the *Oprah Winfrey Show* and identified strongly with her "Remembering the Spirit" segment. My work schedule had certainly precluded watching television. I learned that I share the experience with many in this world who had to learn to rebalance life and to overcome monumental obstacles.

In taking physical inventory, I was minus my left breast. The removal of this barrier would most assuredly mean a better golf swing. That's the only positive thing I could squeak out on that count.

At the end of four months into my nine-month treatment program, I started back to work part time. My employer was agreeable to allowing me to work some of that time from home. The flexibility in this regard was most helpful. I tapped into conference calls each week from home to stay up on all the changes and issues. I worked from my computer, developing new programs, and connecting with my client group via email. And during the intermittent weeks away from chemo, when I felt well enough I went into the office for mornings only. It was not easy to stay out of the stress inherent in a restructuring environment, but it was a good trial run for me and also allowed me to help some people along the way. In the long run, that did a lot of good for my frame of mind.

There are a few little inspirations that I have carried with me throughout life that have helped me to be a positive person. The first one is, "When you look good, you feel good and when you feel good, you do good." Once recovered from my bed rest after surgery, I made it a point to dress as well as I could, to put on my makeup each day, and to use the tips I had learned in the Look Good, Feel Better program. It's not a matter of being a size six model. It's a matter of doing the best with what you have.

When I had completely finished my nine months of treatment, I spent an entire day in my red plaid pajamas, just for the heck of it. It was a deliciously decadent thing to do. Being a sloth for very temporary periods can do wonders for your outlook. You should try it. I also share the famous Mrs. Gump's philosophy, "Life is like a box of chocolates. Ya jist never know what your gonna git." That's what life is all about, so we have to make the best of it. The more we can do it with surprise and wonderment, enjoying every day with new respect and enthusiasm, the more we will receive from the experience of life. Otherwise, it would be a tremendous waste of a very special opportunity.

There are a number of expert theories about a so-called "cancer personality." I am here to tell you from first-hand experience that it is my educated opinion that this is a lot of poo-poo. By now, I have met so many people with cancer, with such completely different personalities and backgrounds, that the thought of a specific cancer personality is utterly bogus to me! I did learn, however, that in thoroughly understanding personality "type" one could learn to deal better with cancer and for that matter, with life. In my work, I have studied Carl Jung's theory of personality types and the resulting measurement system of personality preferences called the Myers-Briggs Type Indicator, or MBTI®[1] for short. We use this system in the workplace for personal and professional development. It was in knowing where I fall in that measure of personality preferences that led me to greater understanding and the discovery of my inner being at a time in my life when I was completely lost. This understanding proved to be invaluable to me throughout my journey, not only in dealing with myself, but also in dealing with others. And it also provided tremendous insight in learning to recalibrate the balance in my life. I'll tell you more about this in a while, because it's a special resource that you can use as well.

I believe that life takes us on different paths for a reason. In my case, I felt like a locomotive flashing hell-bent down the tracks, travelling at the speed of light, when all of a sudden, someone pulled the pin and the tracks shifted sharply into a new direction. I was completely and profoundly disoriented. But now that my treatment program has concluded, I am happy about that new direction. Getting back to life in a healthy and balanced way will be an ongoing, everyday, in-depth study for me. Being positive at the right time and in the right place will continue to be a master tool. I will ensure proper maintenance and care of that tool and if it wears out, I'll be sure to get a new one.

I hope these thoughts are helpful to you. I've decided that when I retire some day, I might be like Lucy from the *Peanuts* comic strip. I might just open my own lemonade stand and charge five cents for consultation on all these insights of mine.

---

[1] MBTI is a registered trademark of Consulting Psychologists Press, Inc., Palo Alto, CA 94303.

Chapter 13

Peeling The Onion

There were specific insights that came to me throughout my journey. Some recurred in my thinking like a distant echo reverberating time and again to capture my attention. I listened inwardly to the unique style in which my personality preferences were helping me to cope and to find my way along the path. And I became aware that all individuals would have their own valuable strengths and also their own blind spots through this challenge, just as they do in everyday life. I witnessed it time and again, interacting with the diversity of guests at the Daffodil Terrace Lodge. There were people of all ages, genders, religious and ethnic backgrounds and occupations. If I was observant, I could clearly see the nuances of "personality type" playing out. This often explained how and why people would choose a certain style to communicate with others regarding their cancer. It determined much of the mechanism an individual would unconsciously use to cope with this heavy blow. And it wasn't happening just with the patients. One could observe the same profiles in the interactions of the medical staff and the approach they would take in relating to us and to each other. Again, I could see it play out in the reactions of my family and friends. The notion of a "cancer personality" disappeared from my thinking.

I am neither a psychiatrist nor a psychologist, but there are things that I have learned in my lifetime that I carry with an inner confidence, a certainty that I am experiencing something significant, and so I share these observations with you on that premise.

I must also tell you that I am a qualified facilitator of Myers-Briggs programs and an experienced, ongoing student of this theory of personality type, both in my professional and personal life and that the insights and observations I am going to tell you about are those of a student who continues to learn. Feel free to test my assumptions.

Once upon a time, actually somewhere around 1920, a Swiss psychiatrist by the name of Carl Jung developed a theory of personality that was so credible and interesting that it has endured to this day as a sound basis for understanding "personality types" in many different life situations. A measurement system was developed and perfected in the years to follow by Katherine Briggs and Isabel Briggs Myers, an American mother and daughter team. They studied and expanded the ideas of Carl Jung's famous theory and applied them to human interaction, fascinated with the possibilities this understanding could bring to the well being of mankind. They developed a simple, but scientifically researched, paper-and-pencil questionnaire that is very effective in helping us to peel the layers of the onion to discover our own unique personality preferences.

The resulting measurement system is called the Myers-Briggs Type Indicator®.

It is used all over the world for the purpose of self-development, career development, relationship counselling, academic counselling, organization development, team building, problem solving, management and leadership training, education and curriculum development, and diversity and multicultural training. If you haven't had the experience of discovering where your own personality preferences fall, I would highly recommend that you take the opportunity to work with a qualified facilitator of the MBTI® instrument (see Resources). This invitation is extended to cancer patients, families supporting those patients, and medical professionals. If you have had this assessment in the past but never thought of applying it to the tremendous challenge of dealing with cancer, I recommend that you get it out again, and get some help in understanding the magical insights that are waiting there for you like guideposts along a darkened and unfamiliar highway.

The MBTI® instrument is a self-reporting mechanism that allows you to cast votes for your unique preferences in given situations. There are more than fifty years of research behind the reliability and validity of the instrument, but in the end, you call the shots in the verification of the outcome. So it's not a matter of someone else *telling* you what personality "type" you are; it is a matter of self-discovery with a professional tour guide along to help you find the right pathways. When you understand the preferences of your own personality type during normal times, it can provide a bridge for you during stressful times—like that of having cancer.

There are four different dimensions considered:[2]

Where do you prefer to focus your energy and attention?

How do you like to take in information and find out about things?

How do you prefer to go about making your decisions?

How do you orient yourself to the outer world?

It needs to be said again. It is a matter of *self-discovery*, personal verification and then lifelong learning to develop one's self to the fullest extent. There are no outcomes of good or bad personality types within the MBTI® instrument. Each is uniquely gifted and special. The added component to understanding this theory is in the richness of insight that the knowledge of personality type brings to us about others.

The key to all of this for me is in discovering the right preference to use in a given life situation. Sometimes that means having to stretch out of my comfort zone to develop dormant potential. Through my illness, it was a matter of finding the right balance for my preferences if they became distorted. Research hypothesizes that there are certain circumstances in life that can encourage an imbalance, such as illness, fatigue, stress, and alcohol and other mind-altering drugs. The first three items listed had crept their way, uninvited, into my agenda: illness, fatigue and stress.

---

[2] Modified and reproduced by special permission of the publisher, Consulting Psychologists Press, Inc., Palo Alto, CA 94303, from *Introduction to Type*, 6th Edition, by Isabel Briggs Myers. Copyright 1998 by Consulting Psychologists Press Inc. All rights reserved. Further reproduction is prohibited without the publisher's written consent.

I've already been clear in saying that my life had become badly out of balance. It became a personal quest to regain this balance as a part of my cancer treatment and also for the purpose of building a happier, healthier life.

So this explains some of how the MBTI® instrument works. One would sort out one's preferences between the four different dimensions, using a carefully constructed questionnaire, casting a vote for one or the other side of the dimensions, *but understanding that we have all components within our personalities to some degree or another.*

The dimensions look like this:[3]

Extraversion		Introversion
Sensing		Intuition
Thinking		Feeling
Judging		Perceiving

The end result yields a personality type. Sometimes this is called a "psychological type." There is potential for interesting differences within just one type. So it has nothing at all to do with pigeonholing or stereotyping. And we each have unique ethnic, educational and religious backgrounds, just to mention a few of the other influences that shape who we are and make us distinct from one another.

As an example, my own preferences are Introversion, Intuition, Thinking and Perceiving. Within the range of my type, my personality preferences bring the added features of Empathetic, Accepting and Tender, which colours my personality in a unique hue from others of my same type. It is not important that you understand the complexities of my own personality but that you see to some degree how it all goes together.

Let me give you a little more background to get a quick understanding of this theory. Perhaps you will be able to recognize some of your own preferences.

---

[3] Modified and reproduced by special permission of the publisher, Consulting Psychologists Press, Inc., Palo Alto, CA 94303, from *Introduction to Type*, 6th Edition, by Isabel Briggs Myers. Copyright 1998 by Consulting Psychologists Press Inc. All rights reserved. Further reproduction is prohibited without the publisher's written consent.

Some features of the psychological preferences could be described as follows:

Extraversion—a preference for turning one's focus outward to people, events, conversations, enjoying many friends, lots of activity.

Introversion—preferring to focus inwardly on thoughts, having time to reflect on one's own, wanting to think things through before offering an opinion, perhaps seldom sharing one's inner thoughts.

Sensing—focusing on facts, details, historical data, preferring to do things in sequential order, realistic, preferring activities that appeal to the senses like cooking, woodworking, gardening and sports.

Intuition—preferring the big picture, that panoramic view I was telling you about, looking into the future rather than the past, seeing possibilities and ideas, having an interest in concepts and theories.

Thinking—a preference for making decisions based on objective views, a high regard for logic, having a sense of justice and fairness.

Feeling—not necessarily emotional, but a preference for making decisions based on maintaining harmony, considering feelings of self and others, putting oneself in the other person's shoes, so to speak.

Judging—not judgmental, but rather showing a preference for keeping things orderly and scheduled, making lists and plans, coming to closure.

Perceiving—preferring to leave one's options open, free flowing, easily adapting to change.

And how does all this apply to my experience with cancer, you ask? And why might you be interested in learning about it?

When dealt with a card that has the potential to change your life forever, or to literally stop your life in its tracks, the equilibrium of your personality will more than likely experience whiplash. This can be true for the cancer patient and also for those close to them. It is a time when hidden and undeveloped aspects of our personality might surface and take over the controls for a time. The more experienced dimensions of our personality seem to mutiny suddenly, leaving us with untrained and inexperienced engineers at the controls. That's a scary prospect, particularly in the face of cancer. At a time when we need them the most, our best allies abandon us. In practitioner circles this concept is known as being "In the Grip."[4]

There can be a different reaction to all this as well. It is known as "Type Under Stress" whereby a component of our personality that has always been a strength to us becomes completely overactive. As the saying goes, "A strength when overused becomes a liability." At any rate, this can have the same unsettling effect of distorting the natural personality alignment that we need.

To illustrate my point, I would ask you to think of a person who carries a natural interest for detail (Sensing), this preference providing a strength in his life, that may possibly lead him to an accountant's occupation. Suddenly, this person becomes stressed or ill and begins to over-use this strength, becoming incessantly picky over irrelevant details until it becomes an obsession and a weakness. Upon snapping out of it, he might say, "I don't know what came over me. I can't imagine what I was thinking." It's a time when one might say or do something that will be regretted the next morning. Apparently this imbalance can last for a moment, an hour or even months. We have all had the experience with the involuntary reaction of speaking out or telling someone off, for example, and then feeling so humiliated for doing so that we wish we could leave town. It's not a matter of losing one's sanity. This happens off and on to each of us throughout our normal every day lives.

Since finding a better balance to my life has been a crucial discovery throughout this journey, it was very helpful to me to use my understanding of personality type to determine just where things were out of kilter. And sometimes, it just provided greater insight into my

---

[4] Modified and reproduced by special permission of the publisher, Consulting Psychologists Press, Inc., Palo Alto, CA 94303; from *Beside Ourselves*, by Naomi L. Quenk. Copyright 1993 by Davies Black Publishing, a division of Consulting Psychologists Press, Inc. All rights reserved. Further reproduction is prohibited without the publisher's written consent.

reactions that I knew were quite all right and would balance themselves when the time was right.

This balance refers to our natural "hierarchy of preferences," or the dynamics that occur when you combine the preferences within a personality. But it is not my intent to bog you down with technical detail here. I recommend that you follow it up on your own in a way that will be meaningful to your own personality.

An example of one situation where things went out of balance for me manifested itself in the overuse of my preference for self-reflection or "introversion." It has nothing much to do with being shy, but rather a natural preference to withdraw within my own thoughts, to have some "down time" from the outer world for reflection, analysis and resting. This is my natural tool to re-energize. It served me well through much of my journey. One is never completely "introverted" or "extraverted." We are all a little of both, but we will have a preference for one over the other in given situations, the clarity of that preference being measured in varying degrees between individuals. I can be very "extraverted" in my professional niche, networking with a wide scope across the entire country, taking the lead on presentations, sharing ideas with others, sometimes carrying the conversation in a group to the point where people wish I would let them get a word in edgewise. But when the evening or the weekend comes and my time is my own, I withdraw within my turtle shell, resting up, enjoying my family and the lack of expectation for avid conversation and "extraverted" activity. My husband is geared much the same way, reflective, often a man of few words and so we find this a comfortable thing between us.

When I became sick with cancer, my "Introversion" took over the wheel. There was a period of many months where I did not want a lot of people to come to visit me. Actually, I didn't want *any* visitors. To have a sudden influx of sympathetic company would have been very unsettling. My grumpy factor found this intrusive and perceived that everyone thought I must be dying—a prospect that quite unnerved me. I didn't much like that. So instead, I gave the word at work that I didn't want any visitors to the hospital or my home and that I would be in touch when I was ready. My relatives and co-workers sent me flowers and cards instead, and that was just the most perfect thing to do—for me. When an "introvert's" preference becomes extreme and he or she decides to withdraw, this can be very difficult for the caregiver or significant other. At a time when those who are close to the cancer patient need most to understand what the person is thinking and feeling, all thoughts are carefully locked away and a distance creeps in making a deep connection with that person very difficult. This can be extremely hard on a caring partner.

If on the other hand, I had a strong preference for "Extraversion," I might have wilted like a plant without water, had there not been an abundance of visitors and phone calls and opportunities to talk the situation through, perhaps over and over again. Another cancer patient I knew expressed his hurt and sadness over the lack of visitors, by saying "Boy, you sure find out who your friends are at a time like this!" Often, those who prefer "Extraversion" work through their problems and their experiences by talking. That's how they get energized. The process can be quite different from that of an "Introverted" preference. But if someone preferring "Extraversion" surprises you and becomes withdrawn and difficult to communicate with, you will know that they may need some "down time" and that they are likely exercising the more "Introverted" dimension of their personality. Not to worry. This is not a bad thing. It may not be a comfortable place for an extended length of time for someone with "Extraverted" preferences. Encouraging them to talk or get out of the house might be just what they need, when the time is right. But don't try to apply the same antidote to someone with a preference for "Introversion" until they have had the opportunity to re-energize.

When my preference for "Introversion" became all consuming, to the point where it was not helpful, I withdrew inside myself with weighty problems that filled my thoughts more and more each day. My logic wasn't operating in proper balance, causing the perspective of the problems to become distorted. That was my least-developed preference surfacing and upsetting my usual strength at logic with the sudden lurch of an abandoned teeter-totter. It was by finding a better balance in that situation that I was able to emerge from the not-so-happy depths of my thoughts to talk with a counsellor. Once I saw my problems floating in the air outside my mind, I felt as though a complete inner realignment had been achieved. My logic (which for me *is* my perspective) returned like a long-lost friend. I resumed my sometimes "Extraverted," most times "Introverted" personality preferences and felt quite settled.

For the occasions when these imbalances surface, I have learned some techniques that work well for my personality type and could work well for others. Through most cancer treatment programs, we are encouraged to begin a journal. I did this in the beginning to keep track of instructions about medication and then later to record unusual symptoms I was having. Then my journal naturally evolved into a diary of thoughts, feelings and emotions. It was a good exercise because I can have difficulty, at times, accessing my feelings. They can bury themselves quite deeply. This can leave me vulnerable, these emotions sneaking up on me months or years later. This seems to happen particularly in crisis situations. I handle the crisis but leave the issues buried.

Expressing my thoughts in my journal helped me to tap into things that I didn't even know were happening inside me. Some days I would just sit with pen in hand or fingers on the keyboard, and my fingers seemed to craft the words of their own doing. Thoughts that I didn't know existed were flowing through me and with them, new perspectives that were so enlightening. Distorted thinking would correct itself. Emotions would surface. Sounds like therapy? "Bleh, bleh, bleh," I would say under any other circumstances. "Let's not think about this." And I would tuck it all away in a drawer somewhere with no intention for spring-cleaning, ever. There were too many places to go, and people to see. Life was too exciting, too full of ideas. But now there was time. The incessant busy chatter in my mind had settled. It was a time for re-sorting, recalibrating, rethinking.

My need to be alone to re-energize is paramount. But when this would go on for too long, my husband would say, "Let's go out for a drive," or "Let's just go for a walk for a few blocks until you are too tired and then we'll come back." His gentle insistence would coax me out of my shell and into the sunshine. Getting those endorphins moving was like a magnificent mind-altering drug that you would never find in any pharmacy or on any black market. What was earlier seen as gray or black with no hope of redemption, became bright and beautiful. What was earlier felt as supreme fatigue, became fresh energy and a happy smile and a re-ordering to the troubles of the world. I was able to move them all from an extra-large size carton to a tiny little box that was most manageable.

When I was ready to talk, the "Extraversion" of talking did me a lot of good. I was ever conscious of not adding extra weight to my family's worries, but there wasn't much that I kept from them. Attending a regular support group did not seem to be a solution for me, but for other people, support groups could be a true life saver. It often occurred to me that people who are alone in the world, single or widowed, would not have the very special support that I was given. What a lonely experience that might be! That's when the Cancer Society steps in to provide support to those who are open to it. How very fortunate I was! In many ways, I had my own support group, through my family and friends. After five months of chemo, I made the transition to living with an entire group of cancer patients at the Daffodil Lodge. And whether I wanted a support group or not, the most natural and subliminal evolution took place through knowing that group of special people. We coached and counselled each other, without anyone pulling a set of chairs into a circle at a pre-ordained time of the week, for group discussion. The bond that grew was phenomenal. I talked a lot with these people. I listened a lot. And little did I know that my support group was encircling me like a beautiful, gentle, morning mist, warmed by the golden glow of the dawning sun.

Before I even became sick, my "Intuition" and "Perceiving" preferences were out of whack for about four years. They had been a strength for me in many ways. My preference for "Intuition" coloured the world as a big bag of ideas, concepts and opportunities. It was like looking at Disney World through the eyes of a small child. There were so many things to learn and to try, so many books to read, so many concepts to understand and to develop. It was wonderful. It still is! But as I said, *a strength when overused becomes a liability.* The excitement of the big picture and the possibilities got totally beyond me. I would buy eight books at a time and try to read them all at once, often wishing I could convert myself into a human scanner, with a capacity to absorb information in seconds. I had wonderful ideas for projects to develop with my work. I could see so many ways that I could make a professional contribution to people's lives. My mind began to overextend itself and so did my body, trying to keep up with the constant kaleidoscope of opportunities and adventures. That's where my preference for "Perceiving" became a "partner in crime." When that preference runs amok, I manufacture an unrealistic need to keep all my options endlessly open, to bring in more and more ideas for consideration until just the right thing strikes me. Closure is something I abhor when in creative mode. Closure and structure are like an oxymoron to my creative process. But when I get too many things going simultaneously for an extended period of time, there I will be— exhausted, burned out, beyond myself. Too much closure and structure can be stress-inducing for me as well, so a happy medium is the end goal. One does need a gestation period for the seeds of ideas to incubate and there is nothing at all wrong with that, as long as you can rein it in at the right time.

So what to do about all of this? Are you like this as well? Or perhaps if life becomes out of balance for you, it is another of your preferences gone wild and causing the disruption. Normal psychological disruptions can come in many and varied forms. For myself, a plan has surfaced. If you look back again on the chart of preference dimensions near the beginning of this chapter, it will make sense to you. Looking back at the descriptions of the preferences, what would your type be? INTP—Introverted, Intuitive (represented by the letter N), Thinking and Perceiving? ISTJ—Introverted, Sensing, Thinking and Judging? ENFP—Extraverted, Intuitive, Feeling, and Perceiving? There are actually sixteen different combinations.

I love my preference for "Intuition." I wouldn't trade it for anything. But I will be learning to stretch to the other side of that dimension to access my less preferred "Sensing" to balance my Intuition in the right situation.

Sensing ——————————————— | - - - - - - - - - - - - - -Intuition

My "Sensing" dimension will say to me, "Now Pat, what can you realistically handle here? Use the KISS principle—Keep It Simple, Stupid." It will remind me to enjoy the present moment.

And I love my preference for "Perceiving." It helps me to handle change, to be easygoing and flexible. There is nothing at all wrong with it, until it gets out of hand. I will stretch to the other side of the dimension and ask my less-preferred "Judging" preference to step in, act as a big sister, get things into a structure and know when to draw my wild creativity to closure: "Okay, time to shut all this down now and make some decisions about what you need here and what you don't, because you can't do everything."

Judging ———————————— | – – – – – – – – – – – – – Perceiving

My "Sensing" dimension will take me out for a walk to get some exercise, to do some weight-bearing exercises at the Good Life Fitness Centre (what a good name!), to build energy, to help me bring my weight issues back under control. It will provide guidance with my preference for "Intuition" *when the time is right*, and it will not allow me to "read just one more book" so that I can become overwhelmed with even more possibilities. My "Sensing" dimension will help to ensure that I keep my body strong so that I can keep up to my "Intuition" and all that creativity I like to think about. I must confess that I don't always *generate* creativity. For the lion's share of the time, I just love to think about it all. But that too can be very tiring and stressful if it runs rampant for too long.

What a valuable resource this has been to restore balance to my crazy but wonderful baby-boomer life.

Chapter **14**

The "Shell Game"

Since *we* have been talking about insights and observations, I want to tell you about some observations that I have made regarding a very pragmatic part of this journey, that being my body—my shell.

There was a point when I would have escaped my body for a song, abandoned it in a heartbeat. It wasn't me. I hated it, and, to make matters worse, it had betrayed me: first by gaining so much weight, and then by introducing this juggernaut of cancer to my life. But through all of this experience, we found each other again, and like the joyous reunion of Peter Pan with his shadow, I slipped back into the shell I had been assigned and decided to take full responsibility for it. However, that didn't happen immediately.

The month of December was my first reprieve at the end of my treatment program. I was still working part time, increasing my hours each week to build back up to going full-tilt. Bruce and I decided to begin enjoying the holiday season on the first of December. Instead of a five-day holiday indulgence, we revelled in chocolates and other good eats for the full thirty days. I must admit I talked him into it. It wasn't hard to do, because he had recently stopped smoking. So I got him at a weak moment to join me in this decadent indulgence. After all, we'd been through a difficult time the past nine months and throwing all caution to the winds seemed logical. It was a conscious decision; we deserved it and we thoroughly enjoyed it.

By January 1st I had gained another eight pounds. I blamed it on the drug I was taking to prevent breast cancer—Tamoxifen. I had heard that one of the side effects could be weight gain. Just what I needed, I thought, subconsciously convinced that somewhere "on high" a decision had been made to ensure I would spend the rest of my life very overweight. Perhaps it was the vanity I had experienced at having a wonderful figure through my thirties. "Pride goeth before a fall," my mother-in-law always used to say. I began to stew about this medication that was on the one hand to keep me safe and on the other hand to make me fatter—at best a Trojan horse! I seemed to be hungrier as each day went by, not realizing that the food I was eating was causing my never-ending hunger. During December, the luscious chocolates filled with the creamiest of truffle centres kept finding their way into our kitchen somehow. They were "to die for." And then, of course, there was the slab of homemade chocolate-covered butter crunch that I ordered from my neighbour across the street each year. We would break it up into small pieces and fill little Christmas sacks for each of the boys and a few relatives and friends. Another couple of slabs the size of a cookie sheet would be broken into delicious morsels sealed carefully in a large cookie tin in the fridge and munched by the whole family (mostly me) as the Christmas holiday approached.

I would eat breakfast and then by ten in the morning in my office at work, I would be taking some preliminary bites of my brown bag lunch; and then of course by two p.m. starvation was setting in. "It must be the medication I'm on," I kept telling myself. And that wasn't the only thing it was doing to me.

How about that Tamoxifen? I was to take this drug for a period of five years. For those of you who are not familiar with Tamoxifen, it blocks the action of estrogen in tumour cells in the breast. It is very appropriate for many people whose breast cancer is estrogen-receptor-positive. At the time of this writing, my oncologist says that it is still considered to be the "gold" of breast cancer prevention therapies, although Arimidex is showing great promise as well. By blocking the estrogen development in the breast, Tamoxifen can be a great ally to preventing breast cancer. One of the side benefits is that it is also very effective in preventing osteoporosis. I like these two-for-one deals! But an annoying problem it has caused for me is a magnification of menopause and sometimes extreme hot flashes. Not exactly a marketable feature!

So let me tell you what I have learned so far on this score: part company with caffeine. Don't drink regular coffee; replace it with decaffeinated coffee. Don't eat chocolate. Don't drink carbonated beverages. Don't drink red wine. And don't eat flaxseed bread. Your constitution may be different from mine, but I will tell you in no uncertain terms that if I dare to do these things, I will be mopping myself off the floor as though someone has just wet me down with a fire hose. If I stay away from these foods, hot flashes are a mere warm glow that is hardly uncomfortable and comes through in momentary waves, completely manageable with layered clothing. I also discovered a magic trick. Perhaps it is well known, but I have never heard anyone mention it. When one of these manageable flashes begins, I just take five slow deep breaths and it cancels out before "warm" becomes "hot"—a nifty trick. This doesn't work if you eat what I call a "trigger food," so don't plan to eat chocolates and then go around breathing deeply. Besides, people will wonder what's gotten into you. As the body adjusts to Tamoxifen over a period of months, the intensity of hot flashes seems to diminish somewhat. I was advised to take the tablet at night before going to bed. That way, the flashing occurs mostly at night while I am asleep and is more minimal during the day. Spouses get the downside of this side effect as well. But they too adjust to the new norm. Note that Tamoxifen is not hormone replacement therapy, but this cartoon by Lynn Johnston from *For Better or For Worse* perfectly illustrates our adjustment to hot flashes.

For Better or For Worse

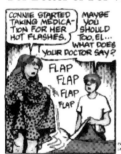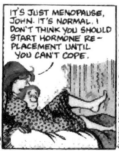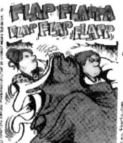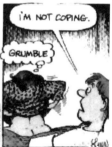

Reprinted with permission from Lynn Johnston Studios.

These byproducts of menopause can be a pain in the "pitooty." However, I've decided that after thirty years of PMS, replacing it with another five years of menopause likely won't kill me. If I had to choose between excruciating menstrual cramps, a grumpy disposition and an aching back every single month, OR the occasional hot flash, I'd opt for the latter. I think that's one of those lemons to lemonade things again. . . .

There was a period, however, where I found my lemonade going completely sour. I would wake up at night, hot and cross, tossing and turning, thumping my pillow, throwing off the covers and lying awake for hours in a state of exasperation. This started to take a toll on my usually good-natured disposition. I began to notice a mild depression drifting into my day and was concerned that yet another feature of menopause was arriving to pull me down. But then I found IT.

Black Cohosh—sounds like something you'd find stuck to the bottom of your shoe or a big ugly snake from a Louisiana bayou. In actual fact, it is the black root of a North American plant. And it is the most effective thing I have found to treat menopausal symptoms— those annoying hot flashes, sleepless nights and low moods. It was once believed to be a phytoestrogen, something that I need to avoid with my estrogen-dependent type of cancer. But the findings now are that it does not have estrogenic properties. It does not stimulate breast tumours. Sounds like a good partner for my Tamoxifen, doesn't it? Apparently it does not interact with other drugs, but should be taken for only six months at a time and then there should be a break. I found it at the drug store, in the herbal section – standardized and certified. I also discussed it with my cancer centre and hope that you will as well, if you are thinking of taking it.

On December 30th, I returned to the cancer centre for a check-up with my radiation oncologist. This was to be the final check on skin reactions from radiation and the seal of approval to return to work full time. The oncologist checked my chest, neck, underarm and abdomen over very carefully, kneading my skin with her fingers inch-by-inch and then listening carefully with her stethoscope. Does cancer make little noises if it inhabits a body? I'm not sure of this, but this part of the check-up with any of my doctors always made me want to smile. "Hello, cancer cells. Are you in there? And what have you been up to?"

I had experienced a couple of startling split-second twinges in my chest over the past month and was curious to ask the doctor about them. She acknowledged that this wasn't unusual—which made my concerns somewhat lighter—and said, "After all, we are all getting older and these little aches and pains are bound to occur." I immediately analyzed between the lines that this was an after-effect of radiation, but since I had experienced these quizzical twinges for a period of not more than thirty seconds over the last month, I determined that if she said so, I could just forget about it. "What *should* I be watching for?" I asked, knowing that cancer recurs for many people and feeling certain that it will for me someday. The doctor looked me straight in the eye and said, "I don't w*ant* you to be w*atching* for anything! Go back to your life, enjoy your family, be happy." I felt an immediate sense of relief but then just to double-check I said, "But I want to know when I have to get to my doctor if there is a recurrence." "If a pain begins and stays—not a pain that comes and goes," she advised. "And the chances that cancer would come back in this area that has been radiated are highly unlikely." I was glad to hear that because I had been told that radiation treatment could be done in a particular area of the body only once.

People at work, and friends in our personal lives would ask, "So are you all better? You look wonderful!" I was conservative in my reply at first, explaining that I couldn't be "cured" of cancer because it was the first recurrence of that small signal eight years before. But I explained that I had the strongest treatment program and that I planned to live a very long time before I would be doing battle again, if ever.

Deep down in my heart, though, I wondered just how long that would truly be.

My doctors were saying *nothing* to give me the slightest lead on this mystery. They were very good at poker faces. I was becoming frustrated about that, but what did I expect? Should I get things in order just in case? Should I be careful to maintain some of that protective bubble I had become so comfortable inside?

And then one afternoon, as I sat at my desk in my office, a question surfaced in my mind, transmitted from a very wise source. "Pat, is this really how you want to spend the rest of your life, with "PENDING" stamped on your forehead?" It didn't matter from which perspective I analyzed this, my answer kept coming up with a resounding "NO." There were just no redeeming benefits to that notion. *That's the day I slipped back inside my body, my not-so-old shell, and decided to become a permanent resident.*

There was much to do. This weight thing was *not* going to win. I had been through a big boxing match with cancer! Surely I could conquer these unwanted pounds that hid my true self under layers of overwork, stress and fatigue. And I refused to return to that constant cycle of exhaustion that I had been trapped in, the past few years. I set a goal to build energy, to shed the chemical experience of the past nine months and to lay the groundwork for many healthy years to come. Dr. Miriam Nelson's book, *Strong Women Stay Slim*, provided all the understanding that I needed, and as a result, strength training became my immediate priority. In the back of my mind I hoped that weight loss would follow, but I didn't want to be discouraged and so I focused on building that storehouse of energy that I needed. The fitness centre was right around the corner from my office. Instead of working away with no coffee breaks or lunch breaks, I resolved to spend my lunch hour at the fitness centre each day. Eventually, this enthusiasm relaxed to a more reasonable three to four times a week.

There were women there of all ages, shapes and sizes. Many were quite elderly, and some were obviously recovering from illness. Then there were the cute little chicks with golden tans and names like Chrissy who were there to get their already fabulous little bodies into even better shape. I learned to use the weight lifting equipment for twenty minutes each time and to build in twenty to thirty minutes of aerobic exercise to my routine. At first it was difficult, but I was encouraged to take it at my own speed. Within a week, I could see that my strength was increasing. I could do eight repetitions of the exercises instead of six and soon it was ten and then the goal of twelve. I hated the aerobic stuff. Sweating and hot flashes—yuck! But I learned very quickly that when I spent fifteen minutes cycling or walking on the treadmill, I would return to work full of energy and enthusiasm. My increased heart rate would jump-start my endorphins, resulting in energy and a grin that wouldn't quit. How wonderful! I didn't fall asleep on the sofa after supper anymore. I felt strong. I felt WELL!

At the end of three months, I still had not lost any weight. I continued to be hungry. I considered writing a book that I would call *The Body That Would Not Lose Weight*. But my strength-training program continued onward. I truly treasured my newly found energy.

I had not received much direction from my doctors about nutrition in light of breast cancer. I knew by osmosis that a low-fat diet, high in veggies and fruit, would be good for me. One sees that everywhere in the news and magazines. It all registered as "yadda-yadda-yadda" to my mind. But my logic was saying that I needed to listen. I thought back to the words of Dr. David Simon (1999), in his book *Return to Wholeness*:

> *"Our bodies are the end products of our experiences and interpretations. To change our bodies, we need to change our experiences. Make a commitment to change your life in the direction of greater love and caring for yourself and those close to you."*

By now, it won't come as a surprise to you that I bought a book called *The Breast Cancer Prevention Diet*, by Dr. Bob Arnot (1999). (I wasn't exaggerating when I said I have bookaholic tendencies.) What a revelation that book was! I learned many things about how nutrition can play a part in preventing cancer. But the key points that finally made their way through the yadda-yaddas and lodged themselves neatly in my brain were in relation to fat cells and regular elimination. Fat cells, particularly in the upper body (where I carried a good deal of excess weight) were estrogen factories! HELLO!

Estrogen factories were not something that I needed at all. Quite the contrary! And not only *that*, a low fibre diet encourages estrogen to be released into the bloodstream instead of being bound by fibre and eliminated from the body—good riddance to bad rubbish, I say! An abundance of fibre in the diet such as fruits, veggies and whole grains, and lots of water, would ensure that estrogen would not be recycled through my body. Dr. Arnot wrote of other things that piqued my interest as well, including the need to reduce the glycemic index in the foods I was eating. The prospect of a Mediterranean diet or an Asian diet being conducive to healthy eating to prevent breast cancer was interesting stuff!

Then one evening Bruce mentioned an article in the newspaper about a diet that originated from France. Diets didn't usually interest either of us. But this was to be a four-week experiment, done by the *National Post* reporter Julia McKinnell. It sounded very successful and we decided to jump into the adventure. Julia's earthy humour added to the bait. The additional feature was that the maintenance diet promised to include red wine and chocolate (if it was 70% cocoa). That sounded like fun.

So we ordered up the book by Michel Montignac, called *Eat Yourself Slim* (1999). As soon as the parcel arrived, I scoured the book looking for the underlying concept to the diet. Thousands of people in France had lost weight using Michel Montignac's method. How could it be *that* effective? I was suspicious that it would be an unhealthy fad diet that would exclude certain food groups, something that I knew would be wrong for my immune system. And the doctor had told Bruce to watch his cholesterol, so we wondered how all this would fit with his needs? When Bruce stopped smoking, he too began to have a problem with weight gain and was feeling troubled about it. He had invested his winter months in long walks to manage his weight and his cholesterol level, but the results were coming slower than he had anticipated.

But sure enough as I read on, the Montignac method was a healthy one, modeled on the Mediterranean diet. And, coincidentally, this diet focused on low glycemic foods to lower the insulin level in the body, similar to what I had read in Dr. Bob Arnot's Breast Cancer Prevention Diet. "Perhaps we're on to something here," I thought. The diet promotes the use of olive oil, lots of veggies and fruits, less high-fat meat, daily yogurt and cheese, lots of water, whole grains and all the things that promote good nutrition. The best thing of all was that I was to eat until I was full. No measuring, or counting or rationing. All right! I could get into this and I wouldn't have to go hungry. We learned to eliminate the high glycemic index foods that were easily replaced with other good things from the same food groups. We learned how to combine particular food groups for best digestion and maximum weight loss.

In the first week, Bruce and I each lost four pounds. In the weeks to follow this tapered off more to a two-pound weight loss each week. Once in a while, a week of no weight loss would occur, then the following week would make up for lost time. But the best news of all is that I stopped feeling ravenously hungry. It seems to me that this came about roughly two weeks into the diet, but it could have been sooner. Cravings for certain foods stopped. When I ate a meal, I was full. Sometimes it didn't occur to me to eat my lunch until two p.m. but I always followed through to ensure good health. At the time of this writing, I have lost thirty pounds and "the body that wouldn't lose weight" is happy to have been adopted and cared for. I will stay on this new approach to nutrition for the rest of my life. Once I achieve the full weight loss that I need, I will switch to the maintenance level and I will never go back to my old habits. Oh, by the way, this change means walking away from sugar. But the craving is gone. That expression "to die for," that so aptly described our chocolate truffles at Christmas, seems quite literally true to me now.

I went for my first haircut one year and one month from the day I started chemotherapy. I looked like a little hedgehog for about four months when my hair first started its new growth. It began as the soft down of a new baby's hair and took some months before it had strengthened into serious hair. When it finally was replenished, it was curly and wavy. I had always had fine straight hair, so this was a real hoot. The additional new feature was that it was steel gray. Gray hair, oh dear! I wasn't ready for that and had it not been for the fact that my husband (and a few others) just loved it gray, I would have coloured it in an instant. So I have decided that I will go about looking younger by losing weight, keeping a very NOW kind of hair cut and dressing in great clothes that are great colours for me. The gray-haired baby boomers are taking over the world, you know.

About a year after my surgery, I finally went to the medical centre to see about buying a boob. The stuffed cottontail from the Cancer Society was starting to get a little pooped-looking and besides, as the day wore on it seemed to climb about three inches higher on my chest than my real boob. I realized that at a management meeting one day when several kind pairs of eyes seemed to be trying not to look at my chest. When I checked inventory later in the ladies' washroom, studying myself in the mirror, it was evident that things were askew. I think I decided to finally get a boob more for everyone else's comfort level than my own.

"What took you so long to come for this?" the prosthetic consultant asked. She pointed out to me that my left shoulder was now lower than my right shoulder because of the imbalance in weight on my chest. (Yes, that Larger Boob syndrome again.) The lady that worked with me was wonderful. She had a small room at the back of the centre that had been carefully decorated like an old-fashioned boudoir. Flowered wallpaper and deep forest-green trim cozied up an otherwise clinical undertaking. There was a large, oval antique mirror standing on the floor for clients to use and broad-brimmed straw hats adorned with flowers decorated the walls. It certainly took the edge off. We tried a number of bras with specially crafted pockets that would hold the prosthesis. I was measured for a size "wow!" No comment. But the measure would have been a hit on the stock market. And don't you dare tell the Troll! The consultant promised that if I lost a lot of weight, my medical plan would cover the cost of a new, SMALLER boob. Another goal, I thought to myself.

There were new things to learn here as well. The prosthesis was filled with some sort of gel that made it squishy like a real breast. "You need to stay away from kittens," she told me. "They get their sharp little claws into your prosthesis and you'll spring a leak." I thought that was hilarious. For people on an economical plan, they could buy the bra with the special pocket and fill the pocket with birdseed. Don't laugh. Some people actually do that. I saved that little story for my husband and he dryly commented that he wouldn't want me to do that in case it attracted the pigeons that make their home outside my office window.

I was to continue to have six-month check-ups for some time. My medical oncologist said he considered mine a high-risk case that needed to be carefully monitored. I finally was successful in pulling that out of him. Each time I would go for my check-up, I thought of the cartoon I had seen of the snowman that was visiting his doctor for his annual checkup. The doctor sat casually on the edge of his desk and addressed the snowman that stood with anticipation in his black top hat and orange carrot nose. Pointing to the snowman's chest, the doctor gave him his test results. "Relax," he said, "those lumps are only coal."

I had come a long, long way from the horror that I originally felt in losing my breast. "Time heals all wounds." "This too shall pass." Isn't it amazing how those sayings always come true? But we are getting a bit ahead of the story and I'd like to tell you more about our actual transition back to the land of the living.

Chapter 15

Phoenix Rising

I was enveloped by the romance and nostalgia of Christmas. Its music played in my ears and wrapped me in the comfort of family and friends. This was my favourite time of the year. My Father Christmas stood costumed in an antique tapestry coat of burgundy and gold, holding his staff and laden satchel, looking down at me from atop the china cabinet. He smiled an all-knowing greeting of good wishes. I smiled back at him.

All procrastination aside, our Christmas tree was finally up. It was adorned with oodles of miniature decorations, each representing to me the memories of my life and family. They were a precious collection that I stored carefully in individual tiny bags, a family heirloom that I had been creating for years. There was the miniature and intricate bird's nest my mother brought to me from her trip to Austria, some twenty-five years ago. The brass viola decoration symbolized one son's love of classical music and his participation as a violist in the symphony orchestra. The tiny mouse in a red sleeping bag and the crisp white figure skate ornament pulled my heartstrings to my late daughter's favourite tree decorations. Memories of her mischievous smile flashed through my mind. The roly-poly teddy bear made from baker's clay was a treasure to my other son. As a little boy, he used to lie on the floor under the tree in the darkness, watching the twinkling lights and colorful ornaments, and dreaming happy thoughts. A tiny clipper ship and a woolly lamb made from hemp rope brought me back to purchases made on holidays in New England with my kindred spirit.

Our Christmas shopping was completed. The shortbread had been baked and eaten up. Requests for a second batch were in. I was delighted to be able to oblige—not too tired, not too sick, not too busy. Boughs of evergreen, nestled with small twinkling lights, wound their way up three sets of banisters on the staircase of our home. In two short weeks the holiday would be here, a time for happiness and relaxing visits, turkey dinners and eggnog.

It was about this time last year that the lump in my breast had surfaced, snuffing my carefree love of this holiday like an extinguished candle flame. I was so sure I would die and not a soul knew of my worries. It seemed so long ago, and at the same time it seemed like yesterday. And now I would find myself a whole year later on the other side of surgery, chemotherapy, and radiation. There were many deep memories behind me, waiting to be packed away into an old trunk of keepsakes in the attic. What I thought I couldn't possibly do, I had done. Where I thought I couldn't possibly go, I had gone.

And I felt so very good. I could read and read without the blur of chemotherapy tampering with my eyesight. I could go for nightly power walks with Bruce and Woody, enjoying the crisp night air and the freedom my body felt as the muscles built strength and energy with each gliding stride. My Echinacea plant was still within me, growing stronger, rooting deeper each day. I could sleep all night long without tubes in my arm to hinder me when I rolled over. I could brush my teeth without the sensitivity that chemo brings to one's mouth. Orange juice and bananas tasted good to me again. My skin no longer complained of dryness and burning and red blotches. My hair was beginning to carpet the top of my scalp like a newborn baby's soft, fine hair. Brushing my hand across the top of my head felt like petting a plush toy. I was still wearing my wig, but pleased at the progress of my natural state. Overall, it felt like being reborn—new skin, new hair, a new immune system, a new life. It was like coming in from an endlessly long walk on a cold rainy day, to be warmed by the fire and fed a steaming, delicious bowl of mulligatawny soup. What a beautiful time of year to emerge from my trials!

I returned to my professional life on a full-time basis. It was a reluctant transition at first. How unusual for my old workaholic personality! I had to ease back in gradually. It was difficult to leave the comfort of spending each day with my husband. Getting back up to the mental and physical pace of the work world required some strategic planning, and I was determined to do it right. My health was uppermost in my mind.

It was so good to see everyone again. I had been in and out on part-time hours over the course of the past nine months, but that didn't allow the usual deep connection with my second family—my colleagues and my clients.

I could see that we had been through parallel ordeals, they and I. They had been facing their own challenge, all the while that I had been climbing my mountain. Restructuring, changes in leadership, tenuous job security, changes in company philosophy, and changes in every policy and procedure known to man had occurred through my absence. "Change" had taken its toll. I thought of the famous television commercial from the web site www.monster.com where people in career transition could go to look for a job. The commercial was effectively done. As I recall, a variety of children seemed to have gained an inner wisdom from studying their parent's experiences about today's world of work. One by one, different voices and different little faces would say something like this:

"When I grow up, I want to file . . . all . . . day . . . long. . . .
I want to claw my way up to middle management. . . .
And be replaced on a whim. . . .
I want to have a brown nose. . . .
Be paid less for doing the same job. . . .
I want to be a yes-man, yes-woman, yes-sir. . . .
I want to be under-appreciated. . . .
I want to be forced into early retirement. . . . "

And on it went. My, how adequately the essence of that commercial captured the mood I was seeing all around me in my workplace!

I gathered folks together one morning and delivered a workshop on dealing with stress during organizational change. We were waiting for some announcements to come from head office at the end of the week. I felt sure that for many, there would be job loss. It was a matter of waiting for the other shoe to drop. Their faces were clearly indicating a lot of sleepless nights. I had learned a lot about dealing with stress these past few months and was glad to share my findings.

One of the exercises we did together was inspired by my personal sessions in learning to relax and maximize my immune system with visualization. I called the exercise "Developing Detached Concern." I recommended it as an approach to my client group in dealing with stressful situations that are beyond one's control, *like that of restructuring—like that of cancer.* The two dilemmas each carry amazing similarities. You might try this as well.

Here's what we did together through part of those agonizing hours of waiting:

Close your eyes. Take five slow and deep breaths. Relax. Imagine yourself climbing up the narrow pathway of a huge mountain. When you get to the top, stop. Take a rest. Lie down on your back and look up at the sky. Take another slow, deep breath. After some peaceful time passes, a beautiful hot air balloon will float down to the mountaintop. Step inside. Feel the balloon begin to gently lift up into the air. Tiny bright stars are blinking against the dark night's sky. Feel the soft wind kiss your face and flutter your hair. Hear the absolute quietness as the balloon makes its way through the sky. Now look down. Scan the universe below you, around you. Feel the connection between your own being and the never-ending universe. Relax. Breath deeply. Enjoy your flight of peaceful detached concern as you observe the world around you.

What is detached concern? This is a technique of living in the present, focusing your attention and your effort on what you are doing at this very moment. You gently detach yourself from looking ahead to the outcome or from looking at the past and what used to be. When you know that the outcome of a given situation is outside your personal circle of influence, there is no requirement to expend priceless energy in trying to control something that you can't. It's like standing on the ocean shore, with water washing up against your ankles and knowing that you can't stop the motion of the waves. Hope for a positive outcome, but focus all your energy into the effort of the immediate task at hand. Acceptance of what *is* becomes vital. Focusing on the moment brings peace of mind and a wonderful ability to concentrate.

I had learned my lessons well in the time I was away from these people. I wanted to share my knowledge. It was not a magic solution, but it seemed to help. I was glad to be back.

Y2K had been the big buildup the past couple of months. With the approaching turn of the century, the experts had been working out all the bugs to ensure that the worldwide network of automated systems would not self-destruct when the date changed from 1999 to 2000. Something about those three little zeroes had become an ominous concern.

For whatever reason, Bruce and I were not worried. Perhaps because of all we had been through together over the past year. From our perspective, Y2K seemed minor. It's interesting how priorities reshuffle when a family goes through cancer together. If the world's computer systems were to crash, we somehow knew we would get through it. It seemed a minor detail.

That morning we had been shopping in our neighbourhood grocery store for a few things to tide us over New Year's Day when all the stores would be closed. The moment we walked through the doorway, the vibes of controlled, constrained panic were evident. Grocery carts were brimming over. People were shopping intently with lists of items that looked more like emergency planning strategies than grocery lists. The shelves that held inventories of bottled water were completely wiped out. Wagonloads carrying new cartons of packaged water were being brought in, no doubt from great storehouses in the back of the building. Checkout counters were stacked with long lineups of people waiting impatiently to get through. Their brows were knit in serious wrinkles of anticipation. A small seed of worry nestled itself into my mind.

New Year's Eve was to be an entirely different proposition this year. It was the Millennium. Like two classic "introverts," my husband and I decided that all we really wanted to do was to keep the celebration simple. We stayed home, sat on our sofa, ate chocolate, drank wine and watched CNN as midnight descended at different points all around the world. We were happier than two toads in a puddle. The world had become a very small place. It was a fascinating experience to be part of.

Each New Year's Eve, when the clock strikes twelve, I find myself wondering what the next year will bring. My thoughts went to this current epidemic of cancer that seems to be consuming mankind. I wondered what the next century would uncover in the treatment and cure of this disease. Will people look back and say, "It wasn't that long ago that we used to cut off women's breasts and fill each person with toxic chemotherapy and expose them to high doses of radiation to ensure they stayed alive!"

"How barbaric!" will say the shocked listeners, knowing that by their medical standards, somewhere off in the future, cancer is a minor concern that can be treated with a one-time pill, a magic bullet that will eradicate the disease. Or perhaps we will step into a machine and replicate ourselves, leaving the old diseased shell behind, to be carefully discarded. I seem to remember looking for that option at the beginning of this adventure.

Actually, the futurists are predicting that in the 21st century, this disease known as cancer may be conquered altogether. The instances of people actually dying from cancer will become fewer and fewer, until it is a rare occurrence. The cancer survival rate has increased from 20% in the 1930s to 50% today. Genetic research will likely discover what turns the cancer cell on and then find a way to turn it off before it even has a chance to make plans. Clinical and screening procedures will advance considerably. The frequency of detecting cancer early enough will dramatically increase and this, in turn, will allow for simple treatment. Biological research will most likely lead us to an anti-tumour vaccine like that used for polio and measles. Did you know that more than 70% of all cancers can be related to personal behaviours and habits such as choosing to smoke, a sedentary lifestyle, an unhealthy diet, consuming too much alcohol or overexposing ourselves to the sun? Since we have the ability to change or control our behaviour, we also have the ability to reduce our risk of cancer.

It will be a good thing when cancer becomes a manageable, treatable illness. That day will come and I suspect it isn't that far off. Sounds like the flu, doesn't it? "Um, excuse me. Do you mind if I take next week off? I just need to get this little cancer thing looked after, and then I'll be back in the saddle next Monday morning." How very different from the eight or nine months of treatment that I have been through. It will happen. I have no doubt. It has already begun.

And what of this talk of "barbaric" treatment? If you have read my story, you will know that this has not been my experience. I feel so grateful to all the people on my medical team, from my family doctor, to my surgeon, to the Victorian Order of Nurses, to my pharmacists, to my social worker, to the nurses who run the Daffodil Terrace Lodge, to my dental oncologist, my medical oncologist, my radiation oncologist and the team of chemo nurses and radiation therapists who support them. I thank them from the bottom of my heart for helping me to continue to enjoy life.

* * *

When we laid our heads on the pillow on New Year's Eve, Bruce sighed a deeply stress-laden breath. Our hot water heater had burst that morning, filling the basement with water. There had been quite a mess to clean up. There were showers to cancel, loads of wash to postpone. There were men to call in to replace the heater. It was quite a production, an upset to our peaceful plans for the upcoming holiday.

"I'm so *tired*," he said to me from his pillow on the other side of the bed. "This last year has been so busy. And now that I know you are going to be all right, everything that we have been through is just beginning to hit me now like a ton of bricks. I'm SO tired!" My heart went out to him. From the very beginning of this whole unexpected adventure with cancer, he had scooped me up, managed his own emotions, taken the reins, held the family together, run the household almost single-handedly, and created the perfect safety net to allow me to find my way. In the middle of all of this, he battled his own challenge to quit smoking after many, many years—a stressful accomplishment. When this man who never complains let me know how he was truly feeling, I knew it was significant. I knew that I was listening to someone who had just been through a terrible crisis, who had operated on adrenalin for nine whole months and was just now coming down. He won't like me sharing this story with you, but I do so for an important reason. We cancer patients and our medical teams need to remember just what the supporting family members go through when they are charged with the daily love and care of someone who is ill with cancer. It is a heavy, heavy responsibility to carry for a very extended period of time. "Care for the caregiver," they call it. Let us not forget.

The low rumble was gradually increasing its intensity. The heavyset mirror on the dresser was shaking and about $6.00 in pennies, nickels, dimes and quarters was vibrating incessantly on the top of the dresser. We awoke to quite a racket at about six a.m. on New Year's Day! We both jumped out of bed in a sleepy stupor and held the dresser. It sounded as though a mega-train was rumbling right down the middle of our street. "Oh my God," I thought. "What now? Maybe I shouldn't have pooh-poohed all the Doomsday Sayers! Maybe the world is going to end after all." And as quickly as it came, the turbulence left us, standing there with our mouths agape and our nerves tensed. Many others reported later that day that they had experienced it too. Some thought the rumble was an early morning snowplow shaking their entire house. Cleaning off the front steps, no doubt? But sure enough, the news reported that we had had an earthquake that measured 5.2 on the Richter scale. It had traveled some 600 miles from its epicentre. Many, having experienced far greater crises, perhaps tornadoes or floods or hurricanes, would laugh at our tension. But this was our very first experience with the unpredictable danger of Mother Nature. Things like this just didn't happen in our part of the world. It was very scary.

And so the new century began at our house.

And what of you? If you were my brother or my sister or my friend, and you told me that you had just been diagnosed with cancer, I would link my arm with yours and give you a hug. Then I would sit you down and I would tell you my story and all the things that I have learned along the way. There were so many discoveries along this journey. It's worth a review. I suggested at the onset of this story that you read with a pencil and paper in hand to collect ideas to pack for your own journey. Let's compare lists. The beginning seems like a good place to start:

1) Stay tuned to your body and pay attention when it tells you that something is wrong. Bodies never lie. Go to your doctor immediately, if not sooner. The earlier they catch your cancer, the less complicated your treatment will be and the greater your chances of survival.

2) Dreams can be your body's unconscious way of notifying you that you need to take action. Be sure to listen.

3) If fear immobilizes you, see a professional such as a social worker, who can help you to do some formal problem solving.

4) Keep your life's priorities in proper balance so that you can live longer and happier.

5) Construct your life such that if you one day ask if you have done all that you possibly could with the mind and the body that you were given, you will be able to answer YES.

6) Remember that life is what happens while you are planning for the future. Don't miss it. Appreciate the present moment.

7) Get a dog or a cat that you can hug. Everyone needs a guardian angel.

8) Find someone you can really talk to—someone who is a good listener.

9) Visit your local Cancer Society office, pick up the free pamphlets; find out how they can help you. *Get educated.*

10) Talk to your health insurance advisor, your doctor, your employer, your banker, or a social worker—find out what financial resources are available to you and then set these issues aside from your worries. *Be proactive on this one.*

11) Remember that the cup is always half full.

12) If you meet any Trolls along the way, adjust your course immediately. Find someone else. Trolls are a very minor part of the professional medical population.

13) Learn about the stages of the healing cycle; understand that you can't bypass them.

14) Be positive only when you are ready to be.

15) Keep your sense of humour when you can. Be silly as often as the opportunity arises.

16) Recognize that it's okay to be sad, to be angry, to be afraid. If you get stuck there for a very extended time, get some professional help.

17) Allow other people to help you.

18) Learn to recognize what is within your control and what is not. You may be pleasantly surprised.

19) You are never alone. Recognize guardian angels when they cross your path. They come in many disguises.

20) Allow yourself the luxury of resting very deeply over a long period of time. Allow your soul to rest along with your body.

21) Ignore statistics.

22) Recognize that your medical doctors may only have time to deal with the physical you because of the sheer volume of patients they are dealing with. You need to explore nutrition and get into cognitive therapy—mind/body medicine. Take the initiative yourself to track down the resources that you will need.

23) Keep your life as stress-free as you possibly can.

24) Ask for what you need from your medical team. Don't suffer in silence thinking that nothing can be done for your discomfort. Sometimes minor changes can alleviate complications you may be having.

25) Have your Myers-Briggs Type Indicator® personality profile done, and most importantly, learn how to apply it.

26) Learn all you can about progressive relaxation. Invite relaxing music into your life on a steady basis.

27) Think of your cancer as a boxing match. You might lose some rounds and win some.

28) Don't let other people's horror stories scare you. Everyone is different.

29) Be a good role model for future cancer patients.

30) Remember that the "caregiver" in your family will need a break now and then, as well as support and encouragement along the way.

31) Reach out to other cancer patients and cherish the relationships that develop. You will share a bond with these people like no other bond you have experienced before.

32) Get out into the fresh air and exercise wherever and whenever possible. Wash your fruit before you eat it. Your mother taught this to you for a reason.

33) Incorporate these new habits into the rest of your ongoing life. Less than 2-10% of malignancies are caused by heredity; 70% are caused by lifestyle; and the vast majority is caused by the complex interaction of genes, environment and lifestyle.

If you are a friend or a family member of someone who is making this journey through cancer, here are some suggestions that may be helpful to you:

1) Be a good listener.

2) Send cards and letters of support until they are well. I loved getting these!

3) Flowers are a nice surprise any time, particularly well into the treatment program when all the flurry and attention has died down and the cancer patient is working hard at staying the course.

4) Test the waters to see if your patient prefers "extraversion or introversion." Some people need their space. Others prefer as much company as possible. And don't be surprised if this fluctuates unpredictably.

5) Try not to say, "Just be positive." Ask instead, "How are you managing?"

6) Help out the caregivers by getting them out for a change of atmosphere or bringing over a casserole (easy on the spices for the chemo patient).

7) Co-workers should feel free to ask how their friend is doing. It is a welcomed question. Don't worry that the subject is taboo.

8) Working with complex details or the slightest physical demands doesn't blend well with chemo. If you are working with someone who is on chemotherapy be conscious of ways that can smooth the edges for your friend.

9) Allowing cancer patients to maintain as much of their normal life as possible goes a long way to maintaining a healthy frame of mind.

10) Do whatever you can to help your friend or family member to stay as stress-free as possible.

After all this advice, I have to tell you again how much I am enjoying getting back to my life. I no longer do multi-tasking at work. I handle one thing at a time. If the phone rings when I am in the middle of something, I ask if I can call back later. I don't take work home with me at night or on weekends. I don't volunteer for everything and spend my time dreaming up all kinds of new projects. I do one thing at a time and I do it well. I now recognize that it's not my responsibility to save the world. There are many other competent people around me who want to help. I no longer stay in the office all day, working away on my computer without coffee breaks or lunch hours. In today's terms, people who can't disconnect from their computers are called "mouse potatoes." I refuse to become one of them. I go out at different intervals and walk in the sunshine and the fresh air. I go for a workout.

As I look down on my garden from my bedroom window, I marvel at the beauty it displays, even in winter. The plants are covered under drifts of snow, but the browned lacy flowers and the crusted frosty foliage peek through the surface to let me know they are still there, sleeping. There are fat lazy snowflakes falling slowly from the sky, settling softly on my garden. I look forward to reacquainting myself this spring with the colours and the special personalities that grow there. I'll be putting in another purple coneflower when the earth thaws and perhaps some new oriental lilies in the fall. Bruce and I may even plant that clematis we've been talking about for five years. I think a deep purple would be very nice.

We will plan to take a trip to see my mother later this year. She will be having her eightieth birthday—a true milestone. And in the fall, I'll be meeting my friends from the Daffodil Terrace Lodge for lunch. It will be good to see them again. Bruce and I might take a trip to Portugal this fall. We have never been to Europe and I may just write a book about our trip someday. . . .

But there I go getting off into the future again. The future is my favourite place. I will *visit* there often, even though I am making a point of *living* in the present moment. That old expression, "today is the first day of the rest of your life" carries deep meaning for me today. I wonder if the person who created that phrase ever experienced breast cancer?

FAVOURITE RESOURCES

VIDEOS, CDS AND TAPES:

Canadian Cancer Society   *Cancer, Confidence & You.* A 26-minute video from the "Look Good, Feel Better" program. Contact "Look Good Feel Better," 5090 Explorer Drive, Suite 510, Mississauga, ON L4W 4T9; or your local Cancer Society office.

Digital Rain Inc.   *Cope with Cancer.* A CD ROM for people recently diagnosed with cancer or living with cancer, and their families and friends. An interactive multimedia program by Digital Rain Inc., 468 Queen Street E., Suite 310, Toronto, Canada M5A 1T7, (416) 947-9449; or your local Cancer Society.

Siegel, Bernie S., M.D.   *Meditations for Overcoming Life's Stresses and Strains & Meditations for Morning and Evening.* A double CD set, 1992. See the Web site www.hayhouse.com

Siegel, Bernie S. M.D.   *Meditations for Enhancing Your Immune System—Strengthen Your Body's Ability to Heal.* A CD, 1993. See the Web site www.hayhouse.com

Siegel, Bernie S. M.D.   *Love, Medicine and Miracles—Lessons Learned About Self-Healing from a Surgeon's Experience with Exceptional Patients.* 1991. An audiotape or book. Published by Harper Collins.

PRODUCTS TO KEEP YOU COMFORTABLE

Dreiturm Kosmetik   Glycerin Silicon Hand Cream Available through most estheticians, or you could order it through L'Image 2000 Esthetic Studio, 325 McKee Drive, North Bay ON, P1B 7Y9 (705) 476-7786; include postage & handling. When your face turns to dehydrated toad skin through chemo treatments, exfoliate and use this cream (for usually oily skin folks – your skin will become unbelievably dry & sensitive as well). I also recommend that this cream be used as a daily prevention (you-know-where) against pain from diarrhea throughout chemotherapy. The 200 ml. size will not be wasted—if treatment is six months buy at least two tubes. It works!

Thursday Plantation — Tea Tree Toothpaste. We found this at our local health food store & feel that it may be the reason that I had little (if any) trouble with mouth sores usually brought on by chemotherapy. Tea Tree oil is a natural antiseptic derived from Australia's Tea Tree.

RECOMMENDED BOOKS

Arnot, Robert, M.D. — *The breast cancer prevention diet.* 1999. Boston: Little, Brown & Company.

Chopra, Deepak, M.D. — *Quantum healing—exploring the frontiers of mind/body medicine.* 1989. New York: Bantam New Age Books.

Chopra, Deepak, M.D. — *Ageless body, timeless mind.* 1993. New York: Harmony Books.

Dollinger, Malin M.D., — *Everyone's guide to cancer therapy—how cancer is diagnosed, treated and managed day to day.* Third Edition. Rosenbaum, E.H., M.D., and Cable, Greg. 1997. Kansas City: Andrews McMeel Publishing.

Montignac, Michel — *Eat yourself slim.* 1999. Boisbriand, Quebec: Prologue Inc.

Myss, Carolyn, Ph.D. — *Anatomy of the spirit—the seven stages of power and healing.* 1996. New York: Three Rivers Press.

Nelson, Miriam E. Ph.D. — *Strong women stay slim.* 1998. New York: Bantam Books.

Porter, Margit Esser	*Hope is contagious: The breast cancer treatment survival handbook.* 1997. New York: Simon & Schuster. This little purse-size book is a wonderful gift for someone with breast cancer. It is a compilation of short clips, insights and ideas from women who have experienced breast cancer, and their one very best tip to share with others. It includes everything from making artificial eyebrows, to herbs that help you sleep, to the benefits of petting your dog.
Simon, David, M.D.	*Return to wholeness: Embracing body, mind and spirit in the face of cancer.* 1999. New York: John Wiley & Sons, Inc. This is a beautifully written book that covers the whole spectrum of cancer therapies from mind/body medicine, to natural healing remedies, to cognitive therapies, chemo, radiation, nutrition, and much more.
Williams, Penelope	*That other place: A personal account of breast cancer.* 1993. Toronto: Dundurn Press. A wonderful, factual book.

MORE ABOUT MYERS-BRIGGS TYPE INDICATOR®

Barger, Nancy J., and Kirby, Linda K.	*Type & change—MBTI® leader's resource guide.* 1997. Palo Alto, California: Consulting Psychologists Press, Inc.
Keirsey, David, and Bates, Marilyn	*Please understand me: Character and temperament types.* 1984. Del Mar, CA: Gnosology Books. This book includes a short-form questionnaire to help you to determine your personality type.
Myers, Isabel Briggs	*Introduction to type.* 6th Edition. 1998. Palo Alto, California: Consulting Psychologists Press, Inc.
Quenk, Naomi L.	*Beside ourselves: Our hidden personalities in everyday life.* 1993. Palo Alto, California: Davies-Black Publishing.

Consulting Psychologists Press, Inc.	3803 E. Bayshore Road, Palo Alto, Calif., 94303. Web site: www.cpp-db.com. Phone: 1-800-624-1765.
Psychometrics Canada Ltd.	Call 1-800-661-5158 to resource a qualified facilitator of the Myers Briggs Type Instrument in your local area.

A Personal Planning Tool

A Personal Planning Tool

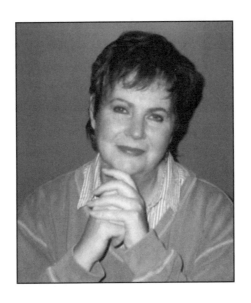

About The Author

Patricia McBain-Roberts is a Certified Human Resources Professional, specializing in organizational development. She lives with her family in North Bay, Ontario. Most recently, Pat is a breast cancer survivor. She is a survivor with a mission to help those who will be affected, either directly or indirectly, by cancer.